GET SLIM AND HEALTHY WITH THE PALEO-DIET

Discover the stone age diet

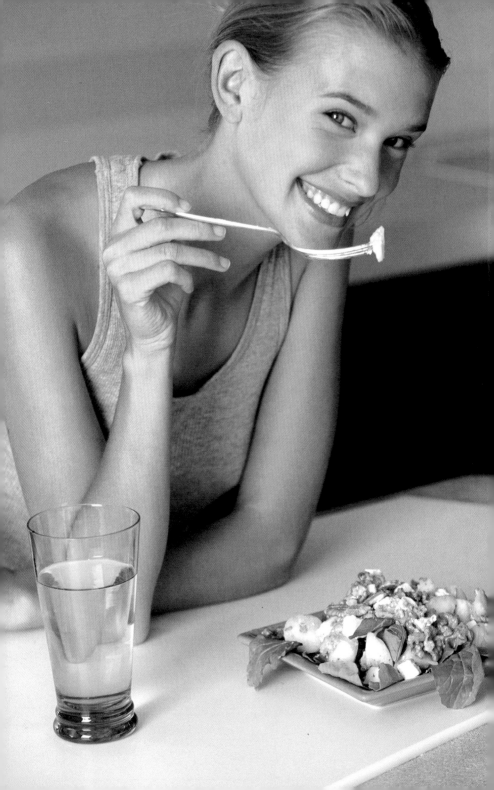

GET SLIM AND HEALTHY WITH THE PALEO-DIET

Discover the stone age diet

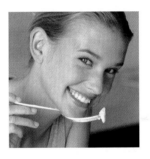

Nancy Cattan

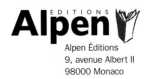

Alpen Éditions
9, avenue Albert II
98000 Monaco

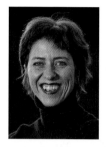

After a career in research of biomedicine, Nancy Cattan, choose to put her knowledge into scientific communication. Doing so, she satisfied her second passion: writing. From an article to another, she approaches with a sharp sense of criticism, subjects which are frequently debated in the medical and scientific actuality. Nutrition is one of her favorite topic and she gives trough this book the kees of a revolutionary and simple diet.

For the present edition
© 2011, Alpen Publishings
9, avenue Albert II
MC - 98000 MONACO
***Tél.** : 00377 97 77 62 10*
***Fax :** 00377 97 77 62 11*

Photo Credits:
Image Source, Photodisc, Scorpius, Goodshoot, Photo Alto, Photosphère, Image State, Creativ Collection, Image Ideas

Printed in Italy
Papergraf press

Introduction

What about to get slimmer by eating what Mother Nature has to offer to us?

Too easy you would answer! Be surprised....

Obesity is increasing. It's not only a concern of rich countries, because it's an obvious fact also in developing countries. This problem is growing so fast, that none of hypothesis studied until now could justify it. Bad habits in our way of living, a food too much rich, a lack of physical exercises, a poor and week genetic, it's probably a mix of every of those things, that could explain a gain of weight, but none of those defects would be the reason of an epidemic.

Epidemic? That's the word! The phenomenon is so gigantic that some scientists came to the conclusion that only a virus could justify such a fast development! Our societies are very confuse towards those problems of weight which are becoming worse despite nutritionals advises gave by great specialists.

Since few years, a new hypothesis as simpler as revolutionary is presented by a nutritionist worldwide known, Loren Cordain (from Colorado University): Man is not genetically adapted to what he is eating. According to Cordain we suffer from being overweight but also from other diseases of civilization, because we do not eat the food matching our body and ours physiological needs. Only a real food revolution could bring us to the road of becoming thin, it's a come back

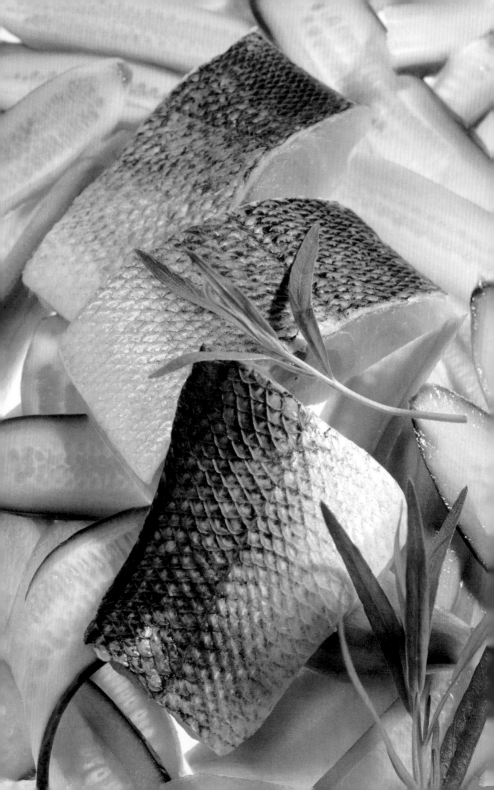

to the origins. Man didn't always eat tagliatelle or crackers and strawberry yogurts… During the most big part of his history, he behaved like a hunter and a picker in others words he had eat what mother nature had plan for him, meat and plants… The main goal of this book is to show you why our modern nourishment is not adapted to our physiology and how you will be able to lose weight by getting closer of the food of our ancestors hunters and pickers.

TABLE OF CONTENTS

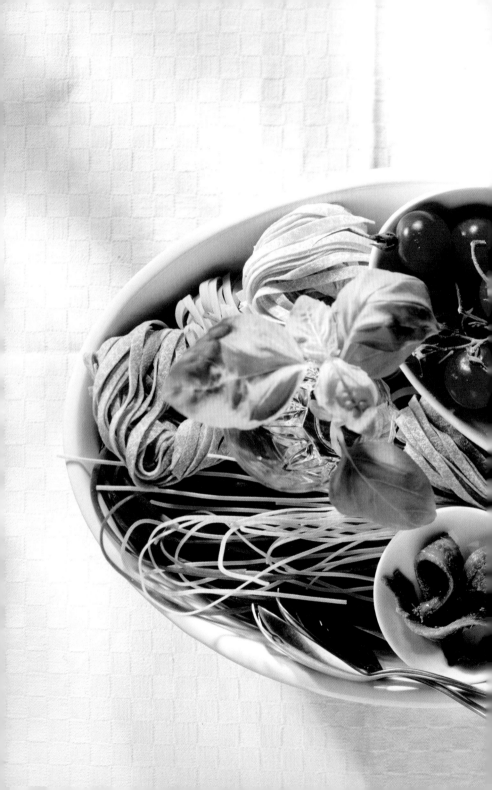

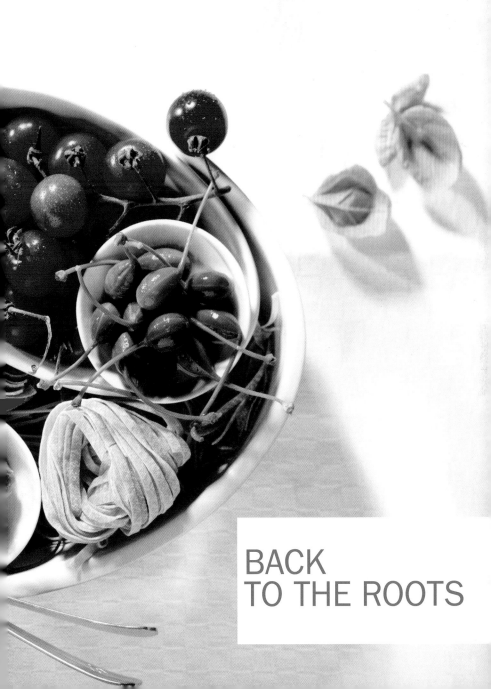

BACK
TO THE ROOTS

BACK
TO THE ROOTS

**He was tall, strong, slim, fit and able to exercise a lot. How do you like that?
Don't look for him around you? He dissapeard for millions years, he was our ancestor. The *homosapiens* otherwise known as "The Cro Magnon man".**

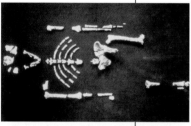

The prehistory starts when the Austarlopithec, appears in Africa 4 million years ago.
Its famous figure was Lucy the woman that the bounds where find during research in Ethiopia.
There are two majors' periods for prehistori-call time: Paleolithic then Neolithic.

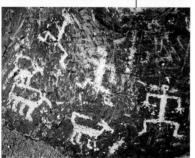

The Paleplithique

The Paleplithique is the longest time of prehistory, the age of the old stone.
Two millions to 12.500 before the Christ.
Man was a nomad then.
His life was outside and in caves.
Several generations of hominids follow each others.
A round 35000 the Neanderthal man step by step will leave place to our direct ances-tor **the Cro Magnon mam**. This guy appears in the Middle East around 100.000 years ago and trusted almost all Europe. He was a master in the sillex cut and he used to produce very sophisticated tool.
He knows how to hunt and to fish very well. He will

draw different kinds of animals in the cave of Lascaux (Dordogne) and the Cave Chauvet (Ardeche).

The frozen age expired around the year 14.000 to 11.000 and the climate became warmer. Bigs mammifers like mammoths went to the big north, smaller types appears, like serfs or rabbits.

Man at that time had to change his way of hunting for that for, he builded the arch... he lives like a predator and make a living through the nature. He moves according the migration of the animals and the growth of the cereals, vegetables and fruits. **He is what we call a "hunter picker"**.

The Neolitical:
the man, became fix

The Neolitical or the age of the smooth stone (from the year 12.500to the age 6000 before Christ0is a big turn in our history. Man is more all over the territory; he went out of the caves and build in some place that he learned to build.

Slowly man is going to live in one only and unique place.

He organizes small villages. He learns to domesticate some animals and how to grow the land.

He knows how to weave and he creates some pottery. He learned also how to stock and to cook the food. He doesn't need to hunt as much as before because he owns goats for the milk and some cheeps for the meat and the woodland lands to grow wheat.

When the man starts to fish...

20.000 to 28.000 years ago the first *Homo sapiens* should have start to eat fish water meat and mollusc. A discovery that was made by American scientists which studied the collagen of the bonds of nine skeleton founded in Europe and in west of Asia dated from Paleolithic up, the analysis shown us that half of proteins digest by *homosapiens* came from red meat. According to the scientists this evolution through alimentary habits more various should have happiest consequences. Eating fish the moderns humans would have come less dependants from fluctuation of the quantity of available meat by developing their sources of food they could assure a growing population.

Cro Magnon was fit and healthy

Like the others mammal the Cro Magnon used to eat whatever mother nature used to offer to him a diet source of nutrishement essentials and various adapted to a lifestyle where physical activity was obliged in order to survive.

Our ancestors had to resist to longs and strong winter time and learn to anticipate period of fasting we had to stock in order to prevent harder periods. To stock the energy as body fat or storages. During a long time in the human nature it was no space for cicada that the winter. A diet source of nourishment essentials and different completely adjusted to a life style where physical activity was obliged to survive. Our ancestors had to resist to longs and hard winters they had to learn how to anticipate terms of no food they had to eat a lot to prevent harder periods to stock the energy either with body fat either with stocks for a long time in the human nature it was no place for cicadas that the winter founded "so sorry". Those who resist where capable to stock during reach periods and to save their energy during poor periods. Economics people in a way.

Health note pad of Cro Magnon

The few fossils discovered and the non secure conservation of bounds to be prudent talking about Paleolithic health. Nevertheless, when we

Cro Magnon didn't have teeth decay

Our so far ancestor picker and hunter of the Paleolithic used to have good healthy teeth, teeth decay appears as man settled and they grow regularly until the 19th century with a bif jump on the 20th century. Then sugar is a product of a first use and it's distributed in the whole world but sugar doesn't explain everything.

What matters are also the few efforts that used to do our ancestors hunters and pickers.

Today our meals are essentially made with soft food and there no muscular effort to do this big to a consequence not enough saliva and more teeth decay.

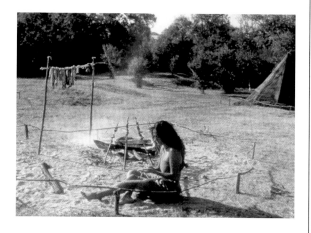

observe the ossements, nustrishments seems to have prevented effects on numerous diseases. The health of *homo sapiens* is generally good and a good nutritional balance: essentialy arthritis on the vertebras, broken, but no gout no osteoporosis neither rachitic due to a lack of vitamin D, neither problems of teeth reflect the "early death". Not so sure the hypothesis that those adults of those days didn't live more than 25 or 30 years sounds to be wrong.

An exaggerate early death

According to Claude Masset a scientist of the CNRS. We went wrong about the hope of living of our prehistorical as ancestors. Infant death was high (half of kids before ten) often attached to infection to small germs themselves existing a long time ago.

Those who riched 20 had probably a hope of living of 35 years, so they used to die around 55 that's mean like the 18 century even with poor hygiene.

The Neolithic: A food heartquick

During the neolitic, the man stopped to be a predator to become a producer. With settlement appear unknown ingredients until then: cereals, diary, sugars and salt.

The Neolithic revolution was born in the Middle east in what we call the fertile half moon .it bring a complete modification of the life style of the societies prehistorical.

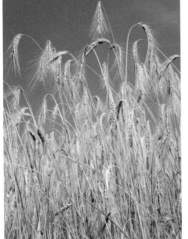

After surviving during ninety percent of his history thank to picking and hunting, man will controls nature under his needs: the vegetal world through culture and the animal world by domestication.

The time of cereals

Million of good grains for the man grow wildly. The give birth to the first cultivated cereals: orge and wheat (engarin, amidonnier, epeautre).

About leguminous plants, they come from bad grass of fields of cereals (peas, vesces, bean, lentil).

The first domestications are also coming from wild race first the cheap coming from the Anatolia mangeon and the goat coming from game, then pork coming from the wild boar then beef coming from the arch.

Bringing meat in the nourishment go lower giving a bigger space to cereals. The quality of the meat changed also because meat coming from the game is fatter than the wild game

By growing animals the dairy products appears in the human food.

The man discovers that salt helps to keep the food in good conditions and he started to like to this nice taste he gives to food.

Gifts of the Neolithic

Ancestor of the famous English porridge, the melted cereals became a kind of king food since the Neolithic time. It's going to give birth to the pancake of dough made by water and cereals then cooked under the fire of the home; this dough cooked by itself in the oven is going to become: **the bread**.

Since then we get used to ferment others products like milk; after few days of fermentation

Milk becomes fix. As it's drain, the curdled can be eaten as is. **It's our cottage!**

The starvation appears

The prehistorians insist that the Paleolithic man is barely missing of food, because he adapts to naturals resources. The big starvation happened during the Neolithic when man gets sedentary and depends to survive of a very few nourishment sources. Essentially the harvests.

Problems appear

The examination of bounds let's know that the firsts farmers just after Paleolithic period were smaller then their ancestors (ten centimeters less). This happened because they used to eat less proteins they had more deseases, more anemia, a lack of iron, a larger osteoporosis, teeth decay and others dentals defects. The food changes are not responsible of those pathologies growing. Anyway all over the world we observed that any time a diet based on cereals was adapted replacing a diet based on hunting and picking, it brings to less hope of living a long and good life.

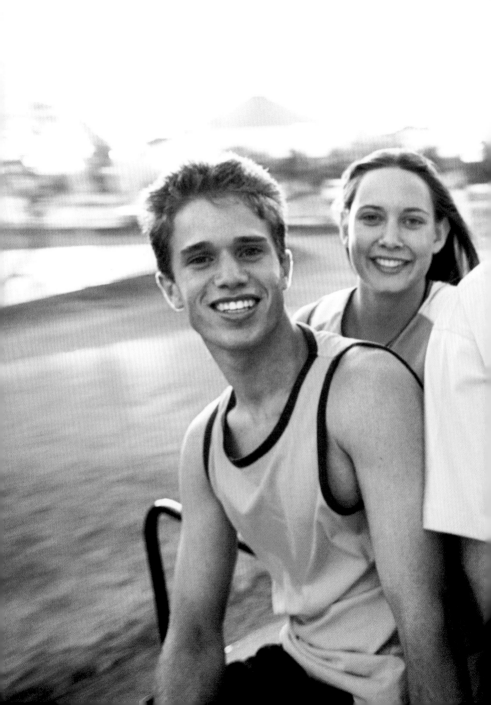

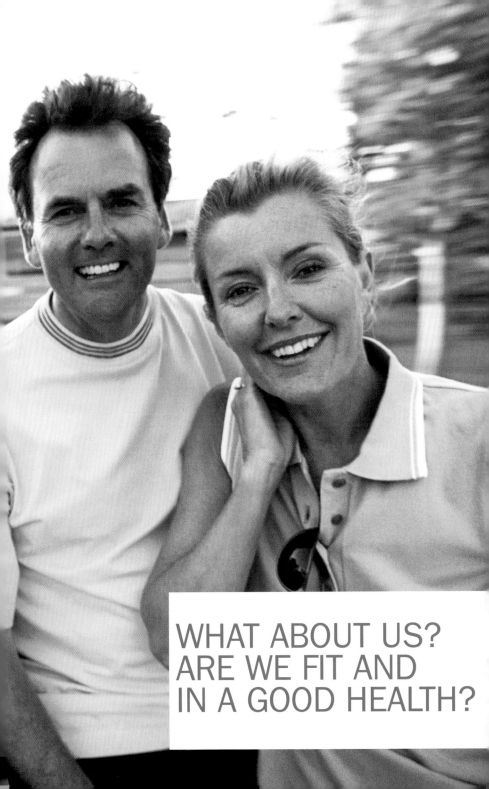

WHAT ABOUT US?
ARE WE FIT AND
IN A GOOD HEALTH?

WHAT ABOUT US? ARE WE FIT AND IN A GOOD HEALTH?

Are we in a better health than our ancestors?

We live longer and longer in developed countries, it's a fact.

But this evolution is essentially related to the progress of hygiene and the end of big epidemic as cholera. This evolution has been helped by the enormous progress of surgery and vaccination. Those both allowed to destroy numerous diseases which used to be dead full.

When we look at it closer the reality of public health is not enjoyable!

New diseases also dead full appear. When disease with infection are going down, "Civilization diseases" are about to explode.

Starting the third century

Our nourishment changed very quickly and recently. Probably too fast.

According to some scientists that would explain our disease of civilization.

The number one: being overweight.

If we think that our direct ancestor: the Man of Cro Magnon appears around 30.000 or 50.000 years, our humankind. Followed during more than **90 % of his history**, the same diet based on wild game of fish and vegetables hunted, fished picked and very soon eaten.

Here we are at the beginning of the third century eating food completely unknown from thousand of generations who came before us.

Nourishment changed very brutally but what about us? We didn't change so much.

Our metabolism looks like very much to the one of our far ancestor of Paleolithic: the man of Cro Magnon.And it's difficult for him to adapt himself to those very particular food created from technology.

First consequence: obesity

The advantage which allowed our ancestors to survive to starvation times returned against us. We are unable to survive to the attraction of food and especially to its variety. Weeat a lot of fat. Sugars we get full of plenty of those moderns products that the food industry show us trough advertising campaign... Products that our metabolism of hunter and picker keep on to switch in fat stocked ugly and nowadays unusefull.

Those ways of eating bring us to obesity, this problem increase slowly in developed countries on the top of that we don't move enough.

Almost 30 % of the French population suffers from being overweight.

The worse is up to come in ten years in France the kids obese aged from 8 to 14 got double...

Let's learn from the past

Without going back to the age of stone diet, based on bodies or insects.

It's seems reasonable to try to get close to them responding to our naturals needs that our genes had always known.

By reducing cereals, the sugar, the salt and a good quantity of diary we will be able to lose weight and also go back to health and the well being.

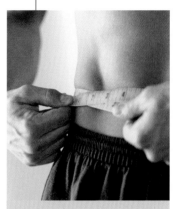

French people are fatter

France has today more than 5,3 millions of adults people obese and 14,4 millions of people being overweight. According to the survey Obepi of 2003 on over 25.000 people over fifteen years old, the French people are bigger and bigger.

Their scale is showing nine hundred grammas more than during the year 2000.

Their waste is also thicker, one centimeter more.

Obesity doesn't stop to grow in all classes of ages.

Since 1997, number of obese increase about five per cent a year.

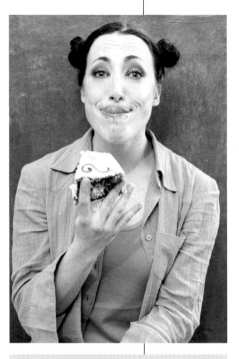

The brain is a control tower of what we eat

The center controlling the hunger is located at the level of hypothalamus. In this zone at the base of the brain together live a center of hunger and a center of satiety.

After receiving all the signals to the desire of eating this is the one which going to decide of our appetite and push us to end the meal or not. Severals neuromediators happened serotonine, neuropeptidey, CRH, galantine. Those are involve in the food and also in the energetic spend.

We eat too much

To get bigger is not coming in one time. Usually the weight settled step by step.

The first step it's called the Dynamic aspect. It's the result of an energetic analysis: we eat more food so more energy than we spend.

The difference doesn't have to be so large in between the two phenomenons to get bigger.

Fifty to two hundred calories a day during a period of time from five to ten years can be enough to gain weight. Usually this weight is going to get stable after.

It's the static step.

Then waves of fluctuation will appear.

Why do we eat more that we need?

We are programmed to eat according to our hunger and not more.

We have psychological, physicals and intellectuals connections which drive our apetite.But very fast we don't know to listen to them. Everything is calling us to eat more and more often.

The industrial food is made according to our hopes that are studied by marketing of those industries.

We are absolutely enabled to resist to those attractive products so likeable with a packaging so pleasant. They are offered to us everywhere; In all companies, at school, in the subway, in each street corner they call us to snack without control which put us in trouble regarding our nourishment balance, it's push us to over eat fat and sweet calories.

Food which maintain the hunger

Most part of animals know spontaneously plan meals balanced and the keep themselves from eating too much. But this balance disappears when food too much sweet or fat is offered. During one month scientists proposed to rats or a portion of water or 5 portions of sweet water until 32 per cent or also one portion of water and 5 of water sweetened. Animals of this group drink much more sweetened water, spend more calories and get fatter more than the others.

The group which had only water is the one who gain less weight. It's seems that it's the same for man and some modern food disturbs appetite signals.

Addicted to snacks

Sodas, chocolate, cookies, all those snacks appear in our daily food true the influence of food industry. Can we become addicted to snacks? The specialist of neurosciences Ann Kelley (university of Wisconsin Madison), think that it's possible. For two weeks she gave to rats food reach in fat and sugar. Result: Such a diet makes mentally the same changes that the one happened with a long use of morphine or heroin. *"The simple exhibition to food with a nice taste is enough to modify the expression of some genes and that's mean that we can become dependent of certain kinds of food (aliments)"* the scientist said.

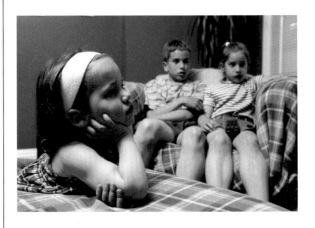

We spend less and less energy

We start to have a sedentary life style, when in fact we are programmed to move. It's like a brutal retirement of a sportsman.

The entrance in an inactive life

We live in a in an environment where food never miss and where the tools of work allow us to reduce and even to skip any physical efforts. But our body is adapted to live in opposite ways. In ways that have been used during all those centuries, then to move was simply useful to survive. The first's victims: The kids. Since last century, kid's weight never stopped to increase despite the diminution of food eaten.

The hypothesis the smarter to explain this paradox is **the larger sedentarily**.

Damage of civilization on the physicals potentiality

A group of scientists watched during several decades, the effects of the Occidentalisation and the settlement on the physicals capacity of an Inuit population. It took only twenty years for those people, who used to have physicals potentiality larger to the Occidentals people, saw their fat increase and their physical power and the capacity of their lungs to go down.

A study about kids living in a suburb of Paris, all of them ten years old, show that more the kids are active less they have fat in their body, even they eat more .But on the opposite way, more they pass time front of television, more the kid had chance to develop fat. The body fat gives information on the "size "of the child. The body fat can be calculated by weight on tall by two (*lire page 53*).

Lights advices!

The recommendations regarding the benefits of to be active don't take care of our potentialities and they are poor and shy; certainly because really nobody cares.

To be close to the global energy spend of our ancestors hunters and pickers, we should increase our spends about seventeen calories every kilo and every day .This is like to run on seventeen kms or walking twenty kms a day, for a person weighting seventy kilos!

Let's forget those objectives, but we reasonably could go above officials recommendations that tells us that *thirty minutes a day of walk on the rhythm of five kilometers an hour,* (a spend of 150 calories), *combine to domestic activity like cleaning* (a spend of six hundred and fifteen calories) *are enough to stay in good shape and health.* Actually when we do those activities we keep on to accumulate more energy then we spend. Of course not in a speed way but regularly until our weight increase silently.

Sport, good for the heart and the arteries

Studies had been done near dockers or students of Harvard, they have been watched with the distance of a half a life. They reveal fact very impressive.

Here we learned that the risk of a first heart attack could be half of it when those people spend 9500 calories a week trough a physical activity coming by an active job or by exercising.

Small comparison

We spend in one day as much as energy that the Cro Magnon man used to do it during his sleep.

We consider that Occidentals people nowadays spend in one day the energy that Prehistoricals people used to spend by resting.

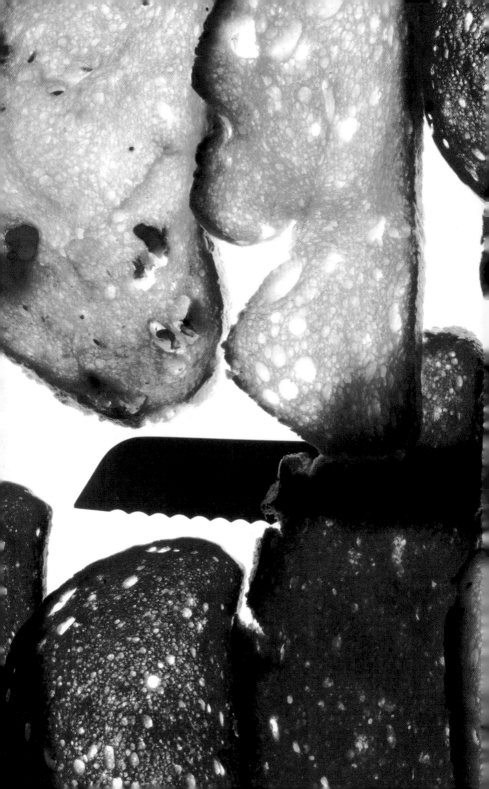

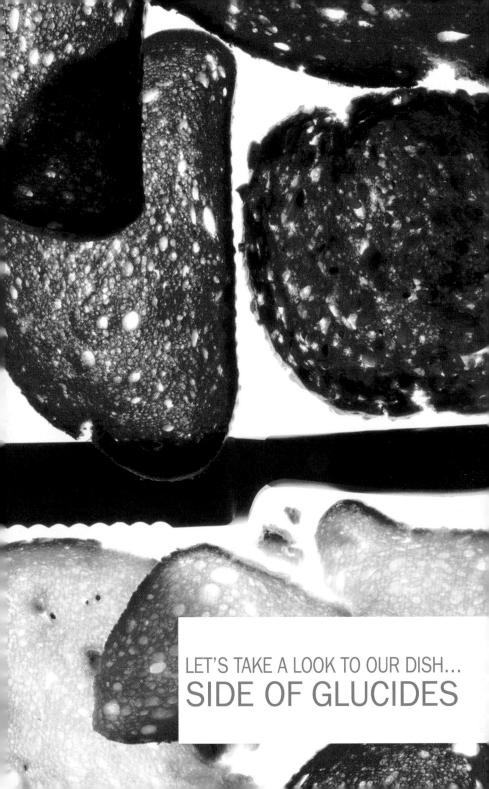

LET'S TAKE A LOOK TO OUR DISH...
SIDE OF GLUCIDES

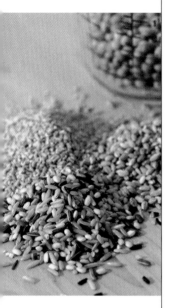

LET'S TAKE A LOOK TO OUR DISH...
THE GLUCIDS SIDE

The glucids are the basis of our nourishment. They cover today 50 to 55%of our energetic needs. Is this justified?

Cereals are modern food!

More or less cereals contain 10% of proteins. Few lipids, **a lot of glucids**, minerals salt and vitamins. We saw it, rafineted cereals, are new aliments to the world-wide scale.

They appear only 10.000 years ago, quickly they became the base of food for humans and they used to represent the best food for a good health.

Now this food is pointed by extremely serious studies. Researches made as well in the USA by scientists like Loren Cordain or in France by doctors like Dr Jean Seignalet, give the same analysis and demonstrate that to eat cereals can bring to several health problems.

A food too rich in cereals and lights products (light in fat but full of bad glucids) could be the cause of **overweight** and even **obesity**.

This kind of food could increase certain **disease cardio vascular** or **diabetes**.

Because they bring too many fibers and stops a good digestion of good products, they might build a deficit of vitamins, minerals salt and oligo elements.

Cereals in numbers

468 million tons of wheat

429 millions tones of corn.

330 millions tones of rice

Are consummate a year in the world.

Eight grains provide 52% of the calories and 47% of the protein consumed in the world.

Cereals, treasurs of antinutritionnels substances and nourishment!

If cereals complete complete contain a good quantity of vitamins (vitamins B), all those vitamins cannot be absorbed by the metabolism because of antinutritionnels substances.

Therefore not even 20% of vitamin B6 (pyridoxine) and the vitamineB8 (biotine) are really absorbed.

Cereals are also very reach in minerals like phosphorus, potassium, magnesium and manganese. They contain also zinc, copper and iron.

But all that is not enough to make them become mineralization food.

First of all, cereals are balanced because they have ten times more phosphorus and five times more magnesium than calcium. And like for vitamins, to absorb a lot of minerals is stopped by anti nutritionals substances like phytates.

Then we have to say that metabolism of the D vitamin (which is an actor of the development of the bounds) is changed by eating too much cereals.

Cereals and autoimmune disease

Some scientists presented the hypothesis that the new proteins bring par the modern food such as milk, cereals or leguminous could disturb the immune system.

Several studies talk about the negative influence of cereals on the evolution of auto immune disease as: rheumatoid arthritis, diabetes, lupus erythematosus, or some disease of the thyroid. According to the authors, cereals bring anti nutritional substances which could modify the bowel wall. The bowel wall will become more permeable to some antigens as proteins of bacteria or virus which will play a starting part in the auto immune disease. In the same time, epidemiological studies tell us that disease auto immune are rare in the population who don't eat cereals.

Meals that increase glucose

The glycemic index, a measure that reveals the fake slows sugars and restore to favor the true ones...

What is the glycemic index?

The glycemic index (IG) of a food gives informations about the blood sugar level (glycemia) of this food. The estimation of it is done by comparison between the pure glucose which is used as a reference with an IG of 100. For example the IG is 43. That's mean 43% of pure glucose.
When the IG of food is high the glycemia goes up. When the g of food is low (<50) it has a lower impact on blood sugar.

Forget about the concept of simple sugars/fast and complexes sugars /slow

This old classification of sugars came from the idea of that more the size of molecule of sugar is small, more it's quickly absorbed and more the glycemia increase brutally.
This conflict between simple sugar and complex sugar has created debate with the notion of index of glycemia. Actually it appears that that potato, corn, white bread and white rice, which are complex glucids that's mean slow, have in fact an IG high; they increase the glycemia faster than the white sugar!
On the contrary, the fructose, a simple sugar, has an index of glycemia extremely low. (IG=20).

What does make move the glycemic index

The index of glycemia of food doesn't depend only from its quantity of glucids **but from several parameters:** the composition of starch, the quantity of fibers, in fat and in albumin and also its superficial structure and the way to prepare it.

For example, a potato cocked in the oven has a IG of 95, the mash potatoes 73, steamed potatoes 63 and potatoes cooked with their skin 57. Other example, green lentils have very few glycemia (IG=25) compare to mash potatoes (73), steamed (73), rice (60), or pasta (50) and this even though the proportion of sugar of all this food is identical (20%).

Meals that increase incredibly the glucose!

If the quantity of glucids eaten by the first men was almost equal to ours, it was also free from the industrial sugars carried by: cane sugar, beets, cereals and dairy products.

Glucids come only from vegetal food (wild plants, roots, nuts, blackberry). Only blackberry and others berries bring simple sugars. The most part of glucids were complex glucids very reach in fibers and then with a poor glycemic level.

Today, we eat too much fast sugars, starchy food and cereals which have a higher glycemic index. **The global IG of our meals increased incredibly** compares to the Paleolithic.

Why the IG of white wheat is higher of IG of whole wheat?

Whole wheat contains more fibers which act like a border: the glucose is liberated less fast into the blood and in a smaller quantity, that's increase the glycemia in a smaller way...

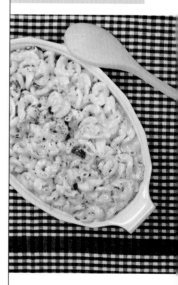

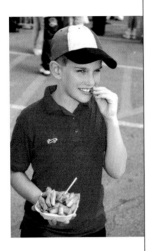

How come the moderns' glucids make us fat?

To understand that, let's travel in the middle of our cells and let's take a look to the kee hormone of energetic metabolism: The insulin. It's the insulin which allowed the cells to use and stock the energy.

The insulin drives the glycemia

We take all our energy from what we eat especially from the sugar. Sugar is a source of energy almost exclusive of the brain and the muscles. But even if it's a vital element, the body doesn't accept big fluctuations of glycemia. The body must adjust its energy intake by maintaining the blood sugar level in strict limits.

• When we eat sugar or food transformed in sugar trough the digestion, like bread, potatoes, pasta or rice, pancreas build immediately **insulin** to allow to use this and to prevent that he stays to long in the blood. Like a kee in a lock, insulin drives the sugar into the cells especially the cells of muscles and adipose tissue.

• But as soon as there is sugar missing (glycemia lower to 0, 8 gram by a litter of blood), the body under the action of another hormone, the glucagon is going to dig in its stock of energy using the glyco-

New concept: The index of insulin

Recently, Janette Brand-Miller, from the University of Sydney (Australia) introduced the idea of an index of insulin of food. It's about to pay attention not to the blood level sugar but to the one more accurate of insulin by comparison with the white bread and this time for an equal quantity of calories (1000). If glycemic index and insulin index cross interfere very often, this concept reveal surprises. The chocolate bar with a high IG obtains a very high score of II (122). But the yogurt with an IG of 62 has a pancreas reaction at least as stronger (II115)! The record is obtained by American candies (jelly beans) which have an II of 160.

gene stocked in the liver and the muscles for its brain and maintaining its stock of fat for the energetic of all other tissues. In the same time, the feeling of hunger starts like an order to rebuild the reserves.

Insulin allows us to stock energy

During a meal the sugar absorbed is used in two ways:

- a part is directly consummate by the brain, the heart, and the muscles...
- too much sugar is stocked at the level of leaver and muscles under the form of glycogen. Then, if the sugar content is still too high insulin make come the glucose inside the fat cells (the adipocytes) and switch it to fat under form of triglycerides. Insulin facilitates the stocking of fat but it stops their destruction.

Leptin is the witness of our excess

Leptin reflect the proposition of fat tissue. Discover in 1994, it's call hormone of satiety. It's acting at the level of the hypothalamus and participates to the control of the food eaten. When the adipose mass is bigger the leptin hidden in the adipose tissue, low the appetite and increase the energetic spend but only in a short term. Obese people have plasmatic levels of leptin around 50 mcg/l when in a person of a regular weight; leptinemia is 5 mcg/l.

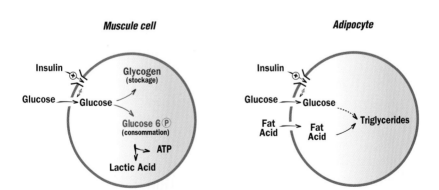

Muscule cell

Insulin
Glucose ——→ Glucose
Glycogen (stockage)
Glucose 6 Ⓟ (consommation)
ATP
Lactic Acid

Adipocyte

Insulin
Glucose ——→ Glucose
Fat Acid → Fat Acid
Triglycerides

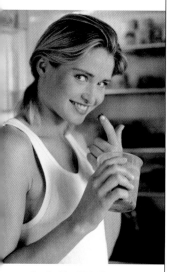

**Food with a high IG
(Base: glucose 100)**

Glucose	100
Oven baked potatoes	95
Sandwich loaf	95
Mash potatoes	90
Honey	90
Cooked carrots	85
Quick rice cooked	85
Corn flakes pop corn	85
Light sugar	75
Watermelon	75
White bread	70
Refined sweet cereals	70
Chocolate bar	70
Boiled potatoes	70
Cookies	70
Corn	70
White rice	70
Beats	65
Banana	60
Jam	55
White pasta	55

The hidden face of insulin

More the glycemic index of food is high, more we have insulin and more we eat!

"The Americans never stopped to low the fat in their food but despite that obesity never stop to develop. This happened may be because they replace fat by those moderns glucids that make higher the blood sugar level." This analysis of Doctor Michael Zermel from the University of Tennessee is based on studies that shown sugars not only made us fat but they stimulate also our appetite.

More the glycemic index is high more we are hungry

Scientists wanted to compare the hunger sensation in a group of obese teenagers after a breakfast and a lunch with a glycemic index or very high or very low. In between meals, some facts permitted to quantify the metabolic and hormonal modifications .The scientists realize that the insulinic answer was clearly higher with meals of an IG high. And the hunger sensation came earlier and the food had been eaten forty five minutes before.

More the glycemic index is high more we eat

Scientists had submitted people to the following experience.
Three different groups of people they had a meal rich in food with IG, high, middle and low.
Then their alimentary attitude had been observed.

No comment about the results!
After a meal rich in food with a high IG, the desire of food was more than **53%** to the one which followed a meal with food of **IG middle** and **81%** when the meal was made of food of a **poor IG**.

Hello Pounds!

To assimilate glucose, pancreas secretes insulin. In "regular" conditions, the quantity of secreted insulin is exactly the same quantity needed to bring down to a regular level the glucose in the blood. Problems start when insulin is demanded in excess. This is the case when we abuse of glucids with IG high during a long period.

We saw it the insulin is the hormone of storage. She brings the sugar in the adipocyte, (the fat cell), then she changes it into fat. The hyper insulin is going to accelerate the process of producing and storing fat from glucose and triglyceride... This brings to put weight on.

Why do we have raging hunger?

When we eat food with a high IG, we create a space for what doctors' call "hypoglycemia reactive". The ingestion of this food creates a higher level of insulin which drives to a brutal fall of the blood sugar level. Then a real sensation of hunger appears. It's the raging hunger! Then we enter into the vicious circle of snacking, which can drive to bulimia.

Food with a low IG

Whole wheat Bread	50
Whole wheat rice	50
Peas	50
Whole wheat cereals without sugar	50
Oatmeal	40
Whole-wheat rye bread	40
Fresh juice fruit without sugar added	40
Whole wheat pasta	40
Red beans	40
Dry peas	35
Whole wheat bread	35
Milk products	35
Dry beans, lentils, and chickpea	30
Whole wheat pasta	30
Fresh fruits	30
Marmalade of fruits without sugar	25
Black chocolate (>60% of cacao)	22
Fructose	20
Soya	15
Groundnut (peanut)	15
Greens vegetables, mushrooms	<15

It was a time we needed to stock in order to survive...

Women are more glutton than men!

Women are more attract than men by sweetened food like cookies, chocolates or milk products very fresh (and very sweetened!).

Men are more found of pasta, potatoes or bread. Result: The part of sugar simples represents 43% of the total glucids for women against "only"39% for men.

Moderns' times are ringing the theory of Darwin

In order to accomplish an evolution, the natural selection plays a part; that's mean that the fact to have certain genes it's an advantage or the opposite. With the human being, the social system, the progress of medicine and others parameters slow down the part of natural selection.

When they couldn't have survive in others times, now people with heredities or dead full illness can have regulars lives and even have kids. We could consider that we reach a point where we are able to go out from the natural mechanism of the evolution.

It's thanks of the insulin that man could survive during those thousands years when the food was limited and the physical activity was intense.

Insulin, the hormone of survivance allowed the man to anticipate on starvation times, imposed by a changeable weather, by facilitating the storage of fat during times of abundance. So when the sources of food became rare, the body could compensate using the energy which has been put on the side. It's possible that the only people able to store enough fat and to spend the less possible could like that survive to the starvation of the poor years.

To survive and to give birth to the men that we are!

What's happens today?

The inheritance that our ancestors left us; this capability to store to prevent rainy days doesn't make any sense now. Today we are facing a food offer drived by a very smart advertising and publicity. We don't eat because we are hungry. Those changes that started as soon as men settled are too recent and have been too quick for us to have the time to get adapted to them. For our genes to adopt those changes, for them to get used to those new consuming habits, we need more than those thousand years that have passed since the development of agriculture and the slow give up of the behavior of the hunter-picker.

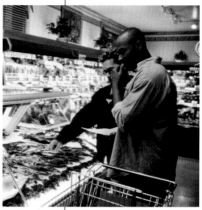

So for the moment, those habits keep on to drive our nutritionals needs and they cannot understand those fines sugars that are the basis of our food.

What are your needs* in energy?

	Age	Weight	Calories
Men	20-40 years old	70 kg	2 700 kcal
Men	41-60 years old	70 kg	2 500 kcal
Women	20-40 years old	60 kg	2 200 kcal
Women	41-60 years old	60 kg	2 000 kcal

*The energy supply recommended according to the sex, the weight and the age. Those values are given for a physical activity called "normal" that's mean it's correspond to the usual activities of the biggest part of the population.

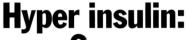

Hyper insulin: Source of a lot of problems

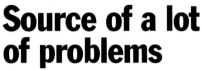

When insulin is called with too much excess, the problems start for your figure and also for your pancreas, your arteries.

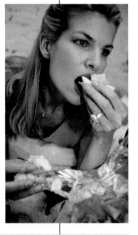

The target is the resistance to insulin and diabetes of type 2

When the hyper insulin becomes structural, the body doesn't react well to the solicitation of the insulin. Cells answer less and less with effectively to this hormone: the sugar stays in the blood. Pancreas is going to produce always more insulin to go over this resistance of the cells, taking the risk to get very tired. Then, diabetes is not so far.

The pancreas cancer

People overweight and not moving a lot have a double risk to develop a pancreas cancer when they eat a lot of starchy food (rice, potatoes and white bread). This is the conclusion of the scientists of Harvard medicine school (USA), who studied the diet of some 89.000 women!

Overweight women and very fund of food with a glycemic index high presents a resistance to insulin which would oblige pancreas to store a big quantity of

Kids: be careful to the diabetes type 2!

Until then, this kind of diabetes happened after 40 years old, to people overweight and even obese. It used to be ignore for kids.

It's not the case anymore.

According to the scientists, the phenomenon is growing in the young Childs especially because infantile obesity explodes in France as well as in others industrials countries. The guilt is pointed on the excess of fat.

The fat cells become slowly more insensitive to insulin. The sugar cannot any more penetrate into the cells; it's accumulating into the blood.

this hormone. Too much of insulin help to develop a pancreas cancer. For women fit and in a good physical condition to eat starchy food has no impact. According to those scientists those results can be applied to men too. In order to reduce the risk of a pancreas cancer, one of the most difficult cancers to cure, scientists ask to people overweight and with no physical activities to replace starchy food by green vegetables, fruits and fibers.

Sugars are worse for arteries than the worse fat!

Foods with a high glycemic index are as bad as the bad fat for the arteries. Doctor Walter Willett, a great scientist of Harvard University (Boston, Massachusetts), started twelve years ago, a big study on the food habits and the way of life of 88.000 women and 40.000 men.

The results obtain show us that to eat food with high glycemic index it's as bad as bad fat for arteries, especially for the people overweight and/or not having a physical activity.

Women who eat more glucids with a high glycemic index (candies, white bread, potatoes) have a coronaries risk two times bigger compare to women who don't eat much of them.

Hyper insulin is going well with...

- Hyper triglyceride,
- Increase of "bad" cholesterol,
- Decrease of "good" cholesterol,
- Hyper blood pressure,
- Hyper urea (too much urea in the blood).

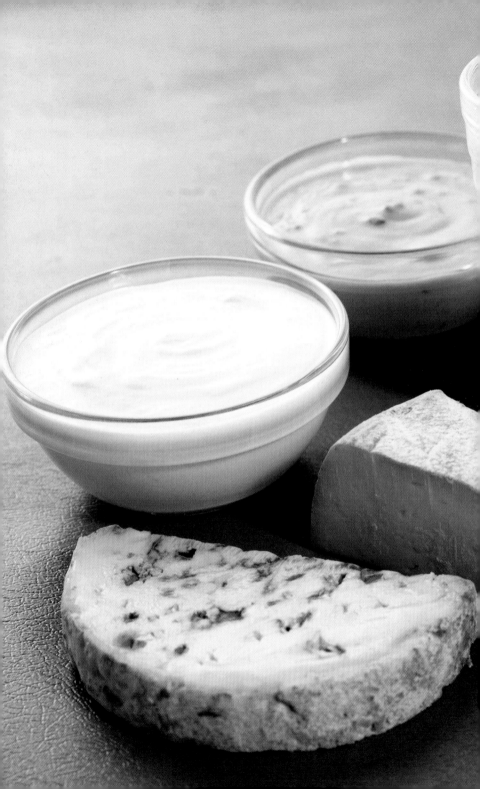

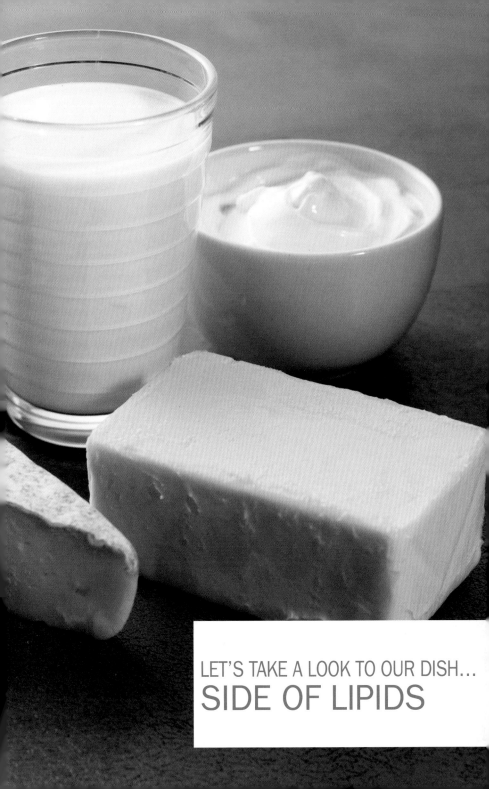

LET'S TAKE A LOOK TO OUR DISH…
SIDE OF LIPIDS

SIDE OF LIPIDS

In a few decades we reduced drastically the quantity of fats in our food. Unfortunately bad fats take over the "good fats".

The different types of fatty acids

We make out fats according the fatty acids that enter in their composition. The fatty acids are chains made essentially of carbon and hydrogen. When fatty acids, because of their chemical aspects, cannot accept hydrogen any more, they are called "saturated". We call them "mono saturated" when they are able to accept only one atom of hydrogen and "poly saturated" when they can fix several of them.

Through fatty acids poly saturated, two of them are essentials. As the body doesn't not know how to produce them, they must absolutely be brought trough food.

They are acids linoleic and alpha-linolenic. Once they are absorbed, both of them turn into others fatty acids. The acid linoleic and the fatty acids that they became are omega-6, the alpha linolenic and all the fatty acids produce by this one are: omega -3.

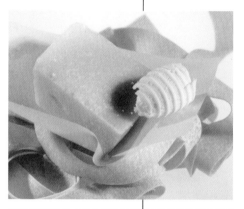

To eliminate fats to slim down it's an absurd idea

The biggest study about our relation between fats and body weight had been done in the USA in the middle of the nineties. In this study, people volunteers had to follow during one year four diets which were different one from each other because of the quantity of fat introduced in each of them. At the end of this experience, the group who had more fats didn't put one gramme more than the group who had taken the poorest diet in fats.

Consumption of fats during the human evolution

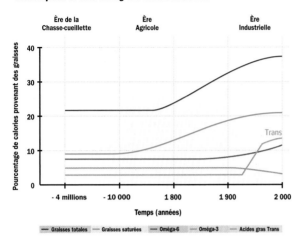

A new thing created by the man: the *Trans* fatty acids

Those fats do not exist as is. The *Trans* fatty acids are produced by hydrogenisation of the oils that pass from a liquid shape to a solid margarine. Our body is unable to metabolize those fatty acids that he doesn't know at all.

All the fats don't have the same value!

With 9 calories (Kcal) a gramme, fats are full of energy. Finger pointed they became the major fear of a lot of people, not only the people who want to lose weight. Tracking down fats and looking to eliminate them from our food we had build heavy unbalance with heavy consequences. It's not the quantity of fat absorbed which is important but actually the type of those fats. As we hunted the cholesterol, we created vegetal oils rich in omega-6 (sunflower, corn, peanut) and we gave up more or less on essentials fatty acids: the omega-3.

The dangers of a diet without fats

With a food without fats, we cannot function well. The kid's brain cannot develop. Diet with no fat at all, reduces dangerously the level of cholesterol global (good and bad) and according to scientists, those diets would create depression, suicid, troubles and hyper activity. Scientists said also that there is a direct connexion between a too law level of cholesterol and the seasonal depression.

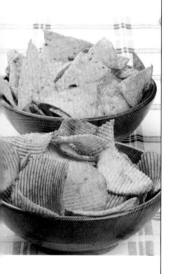

Saturated fat
Trans fats:
A nightmare
for the body

If our body needs saturated fats in a certain proportion, it doesn't care about a type of fat called Trans which represents a real danger for the health and the figure.

Too many saturated fat: hello problems!

The Finland people who absorbed almost 25 % of their calories as saturated fats are facing the worldwide highest level of coronaries mortality. On the opposite this level is lower in Crete where the supply of saturated fats reach note even 8 %.

No comment!

So now we know that the excess of saturated fats is dangerous for health. More than cholesterol in food because it's the supply foods in saturated fats that are going to increase the blood cholesterol, important parameter of cardio vascular risk.

Trans fat and cancer

A famous epidemiologist, Walter Willet (Harvard university, Boston Massachusetts), had follow the food and the health of almost 89.000 nurses. This big survey put the light on the fact that when we eat too much fat it's a risk of cancer. Same thing for the cardio-vascular problems. Looking deeply to those facts, the scientists of Walter Willet's team discovered that, only the women who used margarine and fat food products for cooking (fat products reach in *Trans* fatty acids) have a higher risk of cancer. Numbers are not bigger in the group of women who used to eat butter, eggs, cheese and meat, so actually a lot of saturated fats. But we have to say that the American margarine contains much more *Trans* fats than the French one.

The fatty Trans acids: they are responsible of obesity

The fatty *Trans* acids are the result of transformation of fatty acids unsaturated during the production of margarines, some oils used as seasoning, pastries and different fats products used in the kitchen like solid fat for fried food.

Some studies show us that those fats acids drive adults' people to be overweight. This is not the only side effect... They increase the global level of cholesterol in the blood and the risk of cardiovascular problems.

Learn to avoid them

Infortunatly, food companies are not obliged to explain on the product the level of *Trans* fat. In order to escape from Trans fat, you have to read the list of ingredients. If in this list, there is "vegetal oil partially hydrogen" don't buy it. Don't go neither for margarine with no hydrogen. It would be a bad idea, because usually those margarines contain some oil of palm (around 10 %) which itself contain almost 50 % of fatty saturated acids. (Olive oils, oil of soya, oil of sunflower contain less than 15 %).

The margarine light more expansive than the regular margarine, they contain more than 50 % of water!

Be careful to use with moderation the fatty and solid products for fried food.

Kids are the first's victims

The consumption of *Trans* fats can be incredibly high for some people, especially teenagers.

An article of the *Washington Post* in 1989, described the habits of food of a teen ager who used to eat, 12 smalls brioches and 24 big cookies on a time period of three day. This teen girl used to put into herself 30 grams of *Trans* fat per day and even probably more. Another example the potatoes chips that the teens love. 48% of fats contain in a bag of potatoes chips are *Trans* fats.

So a small bag of chips of 250 grams contains 45 grams of those bad fats. A teen can eat this bag in a few minutes!

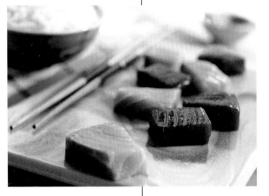

Too much of omega-6 not enough omega-3

Where to find omega-3?

Omega-3 can be find in nuts, colza oil, but also in fats fish like mackerel, salmon, hareng, trout, (tuna, has O-3 too, but it contains mercury too no good for a regular consumption).

Salmon canned often wild, is also an excellent source; the fresh Atlantic salmon, a farmed fish which bring ten times less omega-3 according to a French study edited in 1999. There is very few omega-3 in the meet.

Quantitative ratio omega6/omega3 in the food of

- Eskimos	3/1
- Japanese	3/1
- Cro Magnon man	5/1
- The actual Occidentals people	15/1 à 50/1
- Advised value6	**6/1**

The prehistorical man used to find the two families of fatty acids poly saturated in the physiological proportion of 1 for 1. This ratio went bad after this time. In the Occidental consumption, the ratio is 20 for one in favor of the omega-6.

Why the excess of omega 6 is bad for the figure?

Omega-6 and omega-3 keep a crucial part in our body. They are a part of the membrane of all our cells in an equal proportion. The long chain of omega -3 derivatives determines the fluidity of the membrane. In order to function well, our cells must have a fluid membrane which will permit the receiver like **the insulin receiver** to function in an optimal way. Too many omega -6 will make hard membranes of cells. Those one will become less sensitive to the insulin. On the opposite, a lot of omega -3 will increase the sensivity of the cells to the insulin and will improve the metabolism of sugars.

Why this imbalance?

At the beginning of the last century, the production of consumption oil was small. Oils were cold pressed and we used to buy them in a small quantity, because it was not easy to keep them. The food production increased a lot so the food industry start to push the oils more stable (corn oil, sunflower oil, peanut oil) and refined them. Those oils are the most popular in France, contain only very few omega-3. In the same time, the techniques of intensive farming develop the quantity of omega-6 in a lot of food products. Poultries are feat with corn, cereals reach in omega-6, changing the vision of fatty acids contained in meat and eggs.

Result: usually the ratio omega-6/omega-3in the occidental food is in between 15 and 50 per 1, when it should be between 1 and 6 for 1.

Quantity of omega-3 with a long chain (EPA and DHA) contain in 100 of food

Food	EPA+DHA (g/100 g)
Mackerel	2,50
Salmon	1,80
Hareng	1,60
Tuna	1,60
Pork	0,70
Lamb	0,50
Beef	0,25

EPA: acid eicosapentaenoic
DHA: acid docosahexaenoic

Too much of omega-6 and it's not good for health

When they are processed, the fatty acids from omega-6 develop biologics effects very strong. Some of them facilitate inflammation, tense the vessels and increase the blood pressure or even can low the fluidity of the blood. On the opposite the effects from the omega-3 are much less important. Actually that's mean that an imbalanced diet with fatty acids from omega-6 can be toxic to health. Some studies put under the light a bigger risk of cardio vascular disease and cancers. According to several experts, a return to a food with an equal ratio of omega-6 and omega-3 would have a positive impact on cardiovascular condition of occidental's populations and would reduce the inflammatory disease.

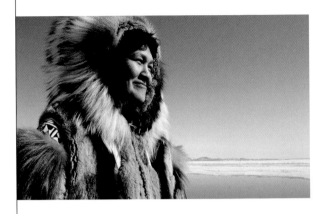

All the benefits of the omega-3

The interest for the omega-3 emerged around twenty years ago when scientists start to think about the health of the Eskimos of the Groenland.

Benefits of the omega-3 for our health

- The omega-3 are essentials for the good development of the retina and the brain of the fetus and the new baby born.
- They low the level of triglycerides when it's too high.
- They prevent from the cardiovascular disease and from some cancers, (breath, and colon, prostate).
- They are anti inflammatory.
- They reduce the risk of depression.

An amazing health. Even if 40 % of their calories come from fats (meat and oil of fish, of seal and of whale), they are protected from cardiovascular disease and some inflammatory disease. We realized very quickly that it was in the nature of those fats rich in omega-3 that was the explanation of this amazing health. Those fats are able to reduce the level of triglycerides in the blood and to fight the inflammatory. This is not the end of the benefits. The omega-3 facilitates a good and harmonious development of the fetus and the infant. Since the childhood, they play a major part in the nervous system.

More omega-3, less coronary thrombosis

A study published in the *New England Journal of Medicine* confirmed that a food rich in fatty acids polyunsaturated omega-3 protect quickly and effectively against coronary thrombosis. During 17 years doctor Christine Albert from the Harvard university (Boston ,Massachusetts) followed 278 men who never suffered from none cardiovascular disease. The scientist observed that the blood concentration of fatty acids omega-3 of the patients was the opposite level of the numbers of death through heart attack. People who used to eat fish at least twice a week, saw, the risk of death reduced of 81 %.The doctor went to the conclusion, that the essentials fatty acids reduce the impact of the troubles of the cardiac rhythm, like ventricular fibrillation and the tachycardia responsible of sudden death.

People with heart problems should consume enough omega-3

The previous chapter had probably alerted those of you readers, that don't like fish. Keep quiet, it's always time to change the benefits of a food rich in omega-3 can be use anytime. The study of Lyon offers the illustration of that. The risk of death of heart conditions people who had a food Mediterranean style with the ideal ratio omega-6/omega-3 had been reduced from 70 % compare to heart conditions people who had a classical diet.

A question of balance

To be healthy, the income of fat has to be composed more or less with a quarter of saturated fats acids, more than half of fat acids monounsaturated and the rest of fat acids polyunsaturated. A target difficult to keep when we take a look on the national food habits.
We will be satisfied with 1/3, 1/3 and 1/3.That will be already good!

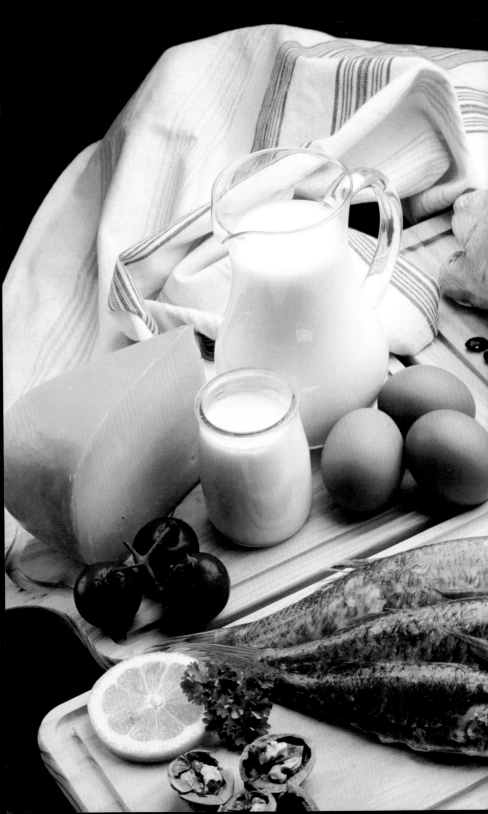

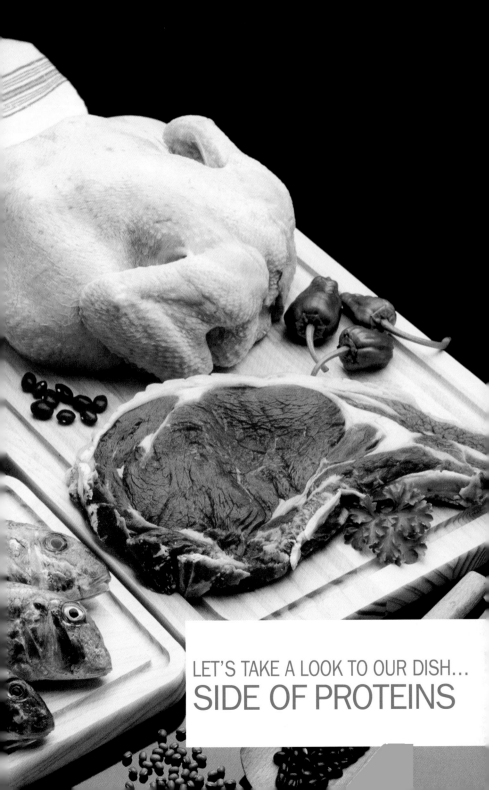

LET'S TAKE A LOOK TO OUR DISH...
SIDE OF PROTEINS

LET'S TAKE A LOOK TO OUR DISH...
SIDE OF PROTEINS

During the times of Paleolithic, the supply of proteins represented between 19 and 35 % of calories and used to come most exclusively from lean meat and fish. With our 10 to 15 % of proteins we are far from this diet and like that we do without component essentials for a lost of weight.

More we have proteins to digest more we spend calories when we rest!

You probably heard about it to lose weight you have to accept to eat less and spend always more energy. But there is a third way more subtitle called "the thermic effect".

What's this magical way? The proteins. This could be a surprise, but by consuming proteins you force your body to spend energy. Much more energy that the one you need to digest sugars or fats.

Result: Your metabolism is boosted.

Not enough proteins put health in danger!

All the people should be aware to have an enough supply of proteins during all their life. Not enough protids can bring different troubles like:
• a smaller muscular mass and also an increase of fat mass
• a general weakness especially from the immune system
• a resistance in a loss in weight

The example to prove it!

A study from the Arizona University had been done with 10 women in a good health condition, between 19 to 22 years old. They had during a day, meals rich in proteins then the next day, meals rich in glucids, in those two meals the portion of fats was small in the two diets. Two hours and half after each meal, scientists took the measure of the thermogenese, that's mean the quantity of burned during a rest. This one was

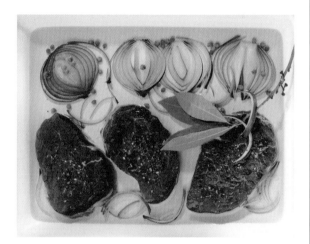

twice important in the diet full of proteins. That's probably the reason why a diet rich in proteins (24 to 30 % of proteins calories) is more efficient on the weight lost than a diet rich in glucids (58 to 60 % of glucids calories).

A study made during 6 months in a group of 65 people overweight, show that the first diet allowed, without caloric restrictions, to lose around 7,5 kilos, when with the second diet, **the lost of weight** is only 5 kilos. 35 % of people who had follow the diet rich in proteins had lost over 10 kilos for 9% in the second group.

Vegetarian diet: a perspective of deficiency!

To eat vegetarian is more developed those days and especially young women eat like that for ethicals or environmental reasons.

Those people are facing very serious health problems related to some deficiency: deficiency of proteins, that vegetal protein (nuts, whole cereals or leguminous) will never cover.

Also a deficiency in iron and vitamin B12 is not good because the nervous system could be damage permanently.

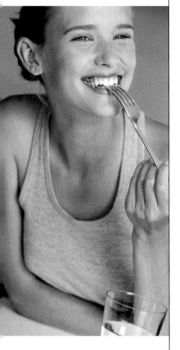

More proteins?
No thanks I'm not hungry any more!

Proteins are nutriments essentials for the loss weight on several points. They help to burn more calories but also they help to reduce the appetite. They also develop sensitivity to insulin and all the metabolism of sugar.

Proteins have also another big quality: they bring satiety. Italians scientists proposed to ten women in a good health condition, three meals with the same supply of calories.

The only difference was one was rich with proteins (68 % of calories),the other rich in glucids (69 % of calories),the last one rich in lipids(70 % of calories). Seven hours after each meal, scientits measure the thermogenese and ask the women about their sensation of satiety. No comment about the result. After a meal

Eating more proteins, bring to have less insulin

Insuline (pmol/l)

- ◆ Régime riche en glucides
- ◆ Régime riche en protéines

Temps (semaines)

Insulin level 2 hours after the meal during a diet of 10 weeks

Eating more proteins we stabilize the glycemia between the meals

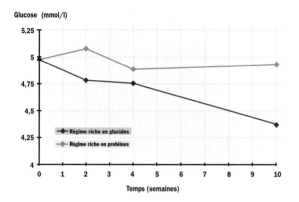

*Glycemia
Between the meals
during a diet of 10 weeks*

rich in proteins, the number of burned calories during a rest time and the sensation of satiety are much higher, so we can see a connexion between the two phenomenons.

Proteins improve the sensitivity of the cells to the insulin

We already saw it, to be overweight bring the cells to be less sensitive to insulin.

The adipocytes full of fat respond less well to the demands of the hormones.

Result: The pancreas has more insulin and when the insulin level is high in the blood (hyperinsulemia), the body becomes storage and that help to put weight on. It's a vicious circle.

During a diet to lose weight, by increasing the supply of proteins and lowering the glucids we have **less insulin** after a meal and also we **stabilize the glycemia** between the meals (graphs).

According to doctor Piatti of the University of Milano (Italy), the cells sensitivity to insulin is much better. Dr Piatti offered to 25 obese women two kinds of low calories diets. The first one contained 45 % of proteins, 35 % of sugars and 20% of fat. The second one had 60 % of glucids, 20% of proteins and 20 % of fat. After three weeks of diet, doctor Piatti came to conclusion that:

The diet rich in proteins improve the insulin sensitivity when the diet rich in glucids had low it.

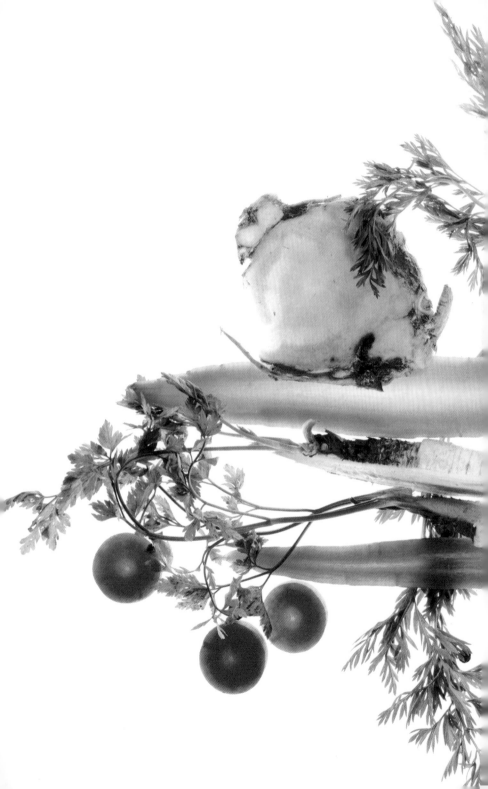

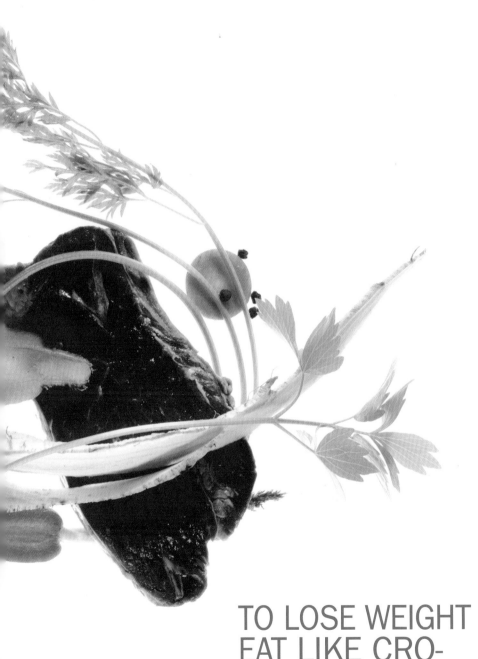

TO LOSE WEIGHT
EAT LIKE CRO-
MAGNON MAN!

TO LOSE WEIGHT EAT LIKE CRO-MAGNON MAN!

A tour guided in the kitchen of our ancestors

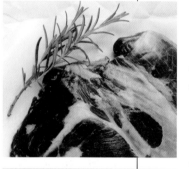

A food healthy and balanced, vitamins and minerals, goods fats... The man of Cro Magnon gives us lessons of dietetics.

Our ancestor didn't eat whatever!

He used to like young game and some parts of meats. He used to prefer: legs, shoulders and head (for the brain and the tong). Parts that he know very well to cut with silex. He loved also snails, reptiles, (lizards, snakes) and insects (grasshopper, caterpillar, verse) all those animal gave him a lot of proteins and a lot of calcium. Would you like some?

Our far ancestor didn't eat when he wanted to eat it. His food, produced by hunting and fishing was under submitted to the climate and his housing conditions.

But when scientists took a look on his dish, they could saw this prehistorical man respected much more than us the recommendations of experts in nutrition.

How the Paleolithic man reach this dietetical performance?

Simply by eating what Mother Nature used to offer to him: game, fruits and wild herbs, various plants, no animal milk (beside maternal milk), some seed and wild cereals?

A distribution of calories very different from the one we have

His diet was composed of 35 % of proteins essentially from animals: almost 3 grams a kilo and a day. The triple of our daily portion!

Fats were more rare with only 22 % of calories (1g per kilo) but especially he used to eat three times less than us saturated fat.

The ratio acids fats unsaturated/acids fats saturated, (which means bad fats /goods fats), was close to the recent recommendations, very far from the modern man, which used to protect him from a lot of pathologies like cardiovascular problems.

His mains sources of fat were meat but also seeds and later in the prehistorical times: fish and seafood.

The supply of glucids was little bit less than the one of today (43% versus 46%) but it was made most exclusively from complexes glucids.

Comparison between Paleolithic food and modern food (By G. Delluc)

	The high Paleolithic	Today
Animal protids	26 %	8 %
Vegetal protids	9 %	4 %
Glucids complexes	42 %	29 %
Glucids simples	1 %	17 %
Animals lipids	9 %	40 %
Vegetal lipids	13 %	2 %
Cholesterol	670 mg/j	480 mg/j
Fibers	100 g/j	15 g/j
Sodium	690 mg/j	2 300-7 000 mg/j

Comparison of distribution of classes of fatty acids at the time of Paleolithic high and today (by B. Eaton)

Fats acids (%)	High Paleolithic	Today
Fatty acids saturated	23,7	45
Monounsaturated	42	42,5
Polyunsaturated	34,3	12,5

The substantive marrow...

Numerous discoveries of broken bounds revealed that Cro Magnon had not enough with the muscle of the game. He used to like almost everything: the bounds marrow, the brain and others similar things very rich in mono unsaturated fats.

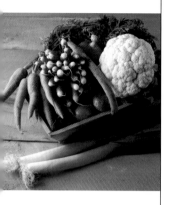

In the daily menu: fibers, vitamins and minerals!

For our Paleoliticals ancestors, no needs to run to the pharmacy looking for vitamins or pills of nutritional supplements.

The food supply in vitamins, minerals and oligo elements were much higher than the daily supply advised today...

Comparison between food supply in vitamins and minerals from the Paleolithic until today

	Paleolithic	France 2000 (Recommended supplies)
Energy (Kcal/d)	3 000	1 800-3 400
Vitamins (mg/d)		
Vitamin B1 (thiamine)	4	1,1-1,8
Vitamin B2 (riboflavin)	6,5	1,5-1,8
Vitamin C (ascorbic acid)	600	110-130
Vitamin B9 (folic acid)	0,4	0,3
Beta-carotene	5,6	2,1
Vitamin E	32,8	12
Minerals (mg/d)		
Iron	87,4	9-35
Zinc	43,4	9-15
Calcium	1 956	900-1 200
Sodium chloride	770	6 000-8 000 (Real supply)
Potassium	10 000	2 500 (Real supply)
Fibers (g/j)	100	25-30 g

A simple reason for that: The picking was almost 70 % of the basis subsidiance. The products of the picking was eaten few hours after they have been picked, often uncooked or with a very few transformation. Trough the countries and the seasons our ancestors used to get delighted themselves with aromatics plants, flowers, young hop, bramble, small holly, fern, wild spinach, nettle, horsetail, dandelion, primula, roots and larges wild berries and differents mushrooms.

Most of those vegetals were richer in fibers and poorest in sugars than the one we know now. This abundant supply of fibers is one of the kee of the Paleolithic health.

Result: our ancestors used to have 3 to 10 times more vitamins then us and quantity of oligo elements higher than the recent supply. Except the sodium and the iodine.

To conclude let's compare this food to the one we have today.

The dish of Cro-Magnon man		The dish of the modern man	
A lot of sugars with a low IG	Good for an energetic metabolism	Too rich in refined sugars	Consequences: obesity and diabetes
Few saturated fats		Too rich in saturated fats	Consequences: obesity with risk cardiovascular
	Good for the heart condition		
A lot of fatty acids unsaturated		Unbalanced in polysaturated Fatty acids, too much omega-6 Not enough omega-3	Bad for the heart
A lot of fibers	Good for the transit And to slim down	Poor in food fibers	That's bring to constipation and then to colorectal cancer
Balanced in sodium Very rich in calcium and Rich in Vitamin C	Good for an activity antiradical Anti oxidant and anti scorbutic	Too rich in sodium	High blood pressure
		Not enough calcium And Vitamin C	Bring to osteoporosis
			Which drive to chronic disease

All that for around 3000 calories a day, which is close to our daily supplies. But also just enough to cover enormous energetic spends! We understand why this ancestor was so fit!

All that for "only" 2400 calories

The benefits of a backward

Here an example of what's happened when man goes far from the food adjusted to his genes

Story of the Aborigine or the misdeeds of civilization

Two hundred years ago, before Europeans colonized it the Australian Continent was occupied by Aborigines peoples, their food way of life was based on hunting-picking. Some tribes still exist until today. The traditional way of life of the Australians aborigines has a high physical activity and a way of eating poor in calories (a lot of fibers, few fats). Those Aborigine that live like that are slim and they ignore resistance to the insulin. On

Consequences of the Occidentalization of the Aborigines

	Hunter-gatherer lifestyle	Western lifestyle
Physical activity	High	Weak
Majors specifications of the diet		
Energetic density	Weak	High
Energetic supply	According to the activity	Excessive
Supply in micro nutriment	High	Weak
Composition in micro nutriment		
Proteins	High	Poor to moderate
- Animals	High	Moderate
- Vegetal	Poor to moderate	Weak
Glucids	Moderate (IG poor)	High (IG High)
- Complexes Glucids	Moderate	Moderate
- Simples Glucids	Weak (honey)	High (saccharine)
- Fibers	High	Weak
Fats	Weak	High
- Vegetal	Weak	Weak
- Animals	Weak (polyunsaturated)	High (saturated)

the opposite way, for those who left the jungle to reach the city, to pass to the Occidental way of life, (less physical activity, diet hyper calorical rich in refined sugars and fats), had a lot of consequences on their health!

A large percentage of the Aborigine population is today obese, suffers from fat diabetes (or diabetes non insulin dependent), intolerance to glucose, hyper tryglicemia, hyper blood pressure and hyper insulin.

A salutary return to the roots

The scientist Karen O'Dea looked closer to this population. She proposed to a small group of Aborigin "Occidentalised" to go back to an ancestral way of life during seven weeks.

To survive from hunting and fishing, doing longs walks in the Australian jungle. Then this doctor saw drastically decrease the metabolism troubles that she noticed at the beginning of the experience (intolerance to glucose, hypercholesterol, hyperinsulin). Those Aborigines had each of them lost 8 kilos. It appears that they eat food poor in calories (1200 Kcal/day), poor in fats (13 %), essentially based on proteins (64 %) - proteins came from wild game a lean meat.

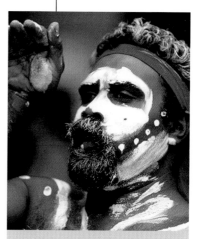

Health report of the Australian Aborigine
(By K.O'DEA)

(a hunter-picker population)
- Good health conditions
- Fit (IMC < 20)
- A low blood pressure
- No increase of IMC and blood pressure as they get older
- A poor glycemia when they starve
- A moderate cholesterol when they starve
- No diabetes no heart disease

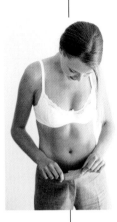

To slim down with the prehistorical diet

The kee of the Paleolithic diet: To control the blood sugar and the insulin.

A terrible diet for rolls of fat

By reducing the portion of glucids in your food (glucids with a low IG),
By eating more proteins (from lean meat),
By finding the right balance with the fatty acids,
You are going to get trade of your pounds especially your fatty pounds.
The ratio glucids /proteins is a major parameter to lose weight and here we are with the efficiency of the Prehistorical diet. Americans scientists demonstrate that a modification of the ratio glucids/proteins of the food we lose weight because we work on the fats stocked.
The muscular mass is preserved.
During a study of a group, 24 women overweighed had followed a diet of 1700 calories per day.
Half of them had a diet rich in glucids. Calories came then from sugar for 55 % (bread, rice, pasta, cereals), 15 % from proteins (around 68 grams a day) and 30 % from Fats, according to nutritionals recommendations of today.
The other group, received food closer to the Paleolithic with 40 % of sugars, 30 % of Proteins (125 grams a day) and always 30 % of fat. After 10 weeks the average loss weight was the same in the two groups (around 7 kilos).

Nothing is forbid for you!

Diets to much restrictive can immediately stop people even before to start.
We have to keep in mind that temporary things have a small impact on health.
What's important is what we do on regular bases.
Time to time to have camembert cheese or Foie gras (fat leaver) will not negatively impact on health if you do follow the diet (a lot of fresh fruits, vegetebles, fish and lean meat) for the balance of the week.

However, women who did the diet rich in proteins lost **6 kilos of fat** and **only 700 grams of muscles**, when the others women who had follow a diet rich in glucids lost 5 kilos of fat and also 1,5 of muscles!

The insulin under control

The Paleolithic diet is based on meals rich in vegetal fibers, in proteins and poor sugars which regulated the level of blood sugar and escape from a bigger insulin answer.

The insulin level running stays moderate.

In a few words: If you have glucids with an IG low, if you eat more proteins and if you balance your food in fatty essentials acids, you improve every metabolism related to insulin.

You store fewer fats, but also you burn more calories and you are lees hungry. With the Paleolithic diet, step by step, you are going to lose weight until you will find your regular weight and you are going to keep it!

More you are going to have weight to lose more the results will be quickly spectacular.

Who has to lose weight?

To know it, it's very simple, there is a magical formula based on high and weight.

We obtain the IMC or index of the corporal mass when you divide your weight (in kilos) by your High (in meters) in square.

That's mean, a person who has a weight of 70 kilos and a high of 1,60 has a IMC of 27,3:

$$IMC = 70 / (1,60 \times 1,60) = 27,3 \text{ kg/m}^2$$

Here is your guide.

• Your IMC is less than 18,5? You are too thin. You must to put weight on.

• Your IMC is between 18,5 and 24,9: You are perfect, don't move!

• Your IMC is between 25 and 29,9: you are chubby. You will have a nicer figure if you lose some pounds.

• Your IMC is between 30 and 34,9: the lights of obesity are on. No discussion you must lose Weight…

• Over 35 you suffer from a severe obesity and over 40 we talk about 'morbid obesity' (a disease). In this case it's very important to be follow by a medical treatment.

This definition doesn't depends on sex or on the age but it's apply exclusively to adults in a good health with a regular size (not high, not to small), not practicing a high level sport.

The case of kids is more complex.

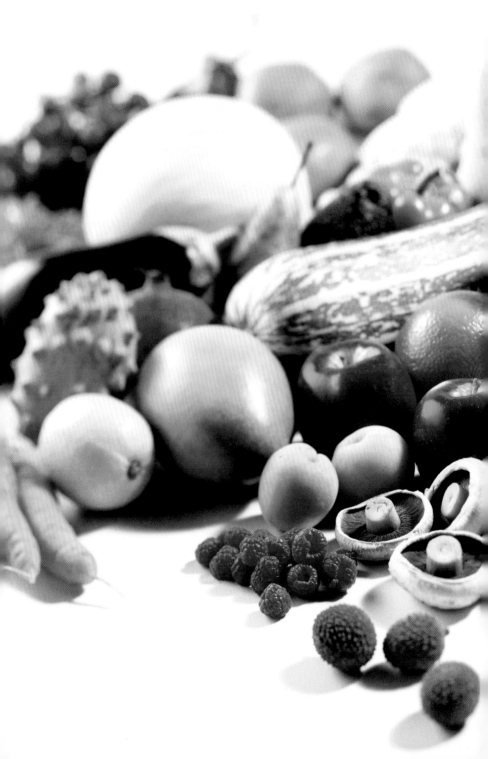

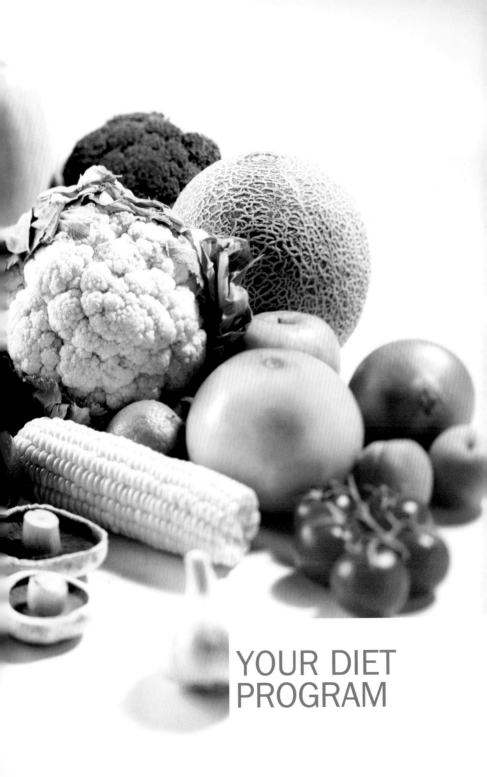

YOUR DIET
PROGRAM

YOUR DIET PROGRAM

Eat more proteins

They make us full, increase the sensitivity of our cells to insulin and they push us to spend more energy. What a shame no to eat them!

Milk : Friend or foe ?

We often think that milk and dairy products are excellent sources of protein. Wrong.

The amount of protein contained in these foods is very much lower than the amount found in fish or meat. In addition, they contain large amounts of saturated fats.

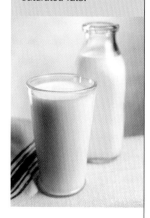

Meats

Meat has a major asset being full of proteins and also in zinc and iron. All meats are not identical. To limit the supplies of fats, choose the white meat much less fat, (we find slices of chicken or turkey with 1 to 2 % of fat and nourished with vegetal food), the game and limit also farm meat too rich in saturated fats. If you eat some take off the fat before the cooking.

• **Red meat**

Beef (rumsteack, slices roasted, sirloin to grill, beef stew, cheek to broil), buffalo, roe deer, horse, wild boar. Be careful: As the horse meat is very fragile it could be infected by some germs in the air.

- You are a man and you are less than 18 years old, you are a woman less than 50: eat red meat 4 to 5 times a week.

- You are a woman over 50 or a man over 18, two meals with meat a week.

Why those differences? because the needs in iron are higher before 18 years old for man and woman and also for the woman between puberty and menopause.

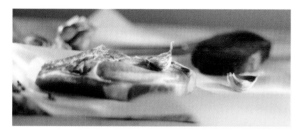

• White meat

Poultry, rabbit, veal (choose a grazer calf whose flesh is darker and particularly tasty). Eat white meat 2-3 times per week.

Origin	Energy kcal/100g	Protein g/100g	Fat g/100g
Wild game			
Reindeer	127	21,8	3,8
Bison	105	26,4	2,8
Horse	110	21	2
Deer	120	20	4
Boar	110	22	2
Rabbit	133	22	5
Duck	126	22	4
Fish			
Salmon	203	22	12,4
Trout	96	19,2	2,1
Livestock			
Beef	289	17,2	10-25
Lamb/Mutton	235	18	15-20
Pork	275	16,7	15-25

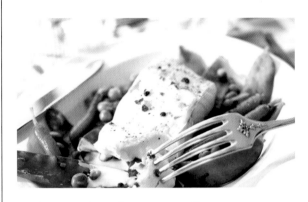

Seafood can be "all you can eat"

- **Lean Fish:** hake, bream, cod, perch, skate, mullet, sole, yellow fin tuna, trout.
- **Fatty fish:** mackerel, sardines, salmon, herring, carp, eel.
- **Crustaceans, mollusks and shellfish.**

Eat lean fish at least 2 times a week, oily fish 3 times a week, seafood 1-2 times per week.

Eggs

Eggs from hens raised outdoors and if possible with flaxseed, 3 or 4 per week.

Reconciliation with offal

They have a bad reputation as today, but offals are full of essentials things. Leaver is especially recommended fort its supplies in minerals salts, oligo elements (iron) and vitamins (A, B9). The veal leaver is of course more tasty but also more expansive. Leavers of heifer, lamb and poultry are much less expansive.

Be careful: the leaver, especially the poultry leaver can contains left over of Drugs (medicine) antibiotics for example. It's better to have leaver from animal raised outside.

You can have some twice a week.

What about cooking time?

Until the Paleolithic high, our ancestors used to eat raw. The use of the fire to cook the food become general before the Neolithic. To cook food is not as usual as it seems.

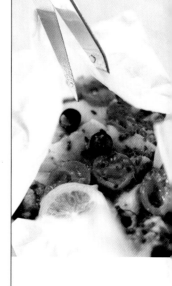

Some techniques of transformation and preparation of products, with a high temperature, could have a bad impact on health. **Barbecues** and **fried food** contain some substances with a potential of cancer (especially for the intestine and pancreas), but also toxics substances (free radicals in particular).
For each type of fat there is a specific temperature, over which there are toxics products.

Some tips come from those facts:

• To use non adhesive kitchen equipment (pan, casserole, pressure cooker) which allow to cook with a few and even no fat.

• For the cooking in the oven: protect the food with tinfoil, without to add fats (for a roast meat oil lightly, for a chicken or a fish their own oil will be enough).

• To avoid the grill (like the barbecue) where the food are in contact with the smoke and the fat of it falls. Give the preference to verticals grills.

• To avoid to eat meat too much cooked (over grilled) and its cooked juice.

• Avoid absolutely fry food.

We must think about a slow cooking of the foods, by using some ways of cooking: with water, steam, double boiler, stuffed, micro waves where the temperature is 100 to 130 degrees C.

Which proteins to use?

It's possible to live without meat. But to live without proteins is a catastrophe.

At the opposite of stored fats, the stored proteins of your body are very weak. Your organism needs a regular supply in proteins all along the day.

Vegetal sources of proteins

All vegetal contains proteins except fruits, but vegetal proteins are not "complete', that's means they are deficient in some amino acids. This next panel gives the idea of the abundance in proteins of several foods and also the chemical index of those proteins.

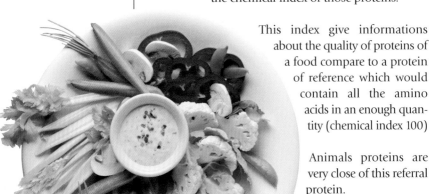

This index give informations about the quality of proteins of a food compare to a protein of reference which would contain all the amino acids in an enough quantity (chemical index 100)

Animals proteins are very close of this referral protein.
A chemical index of 40 means that amino acids of the protein are absorbed to 40 %; the rest is rejected by

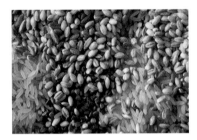

the body. The amino acid deficient stopps the absorption of others amino acids.

• If you are vegan, **each day, eat a different protein source** to provide for your body all the amino acids it needs.

• If you are milk-egg-vegetarian, the milk products and eggs give, in enough quantity, the missing amino acids.

Quantity of proteins and chemical index of vegetarian foods

Foods	Proteins (%)	Chemical index
Almonds	21,26	48
Oats	16,89	71
Peanuts	25,80	62
Mushrooms	2,90	94
Flour of whole wheat	13,70	48
Wholegrain buckweat	12,62	88
Flour of barley	10,50	64
Cheese	20-30	100-125
Seeds of wheat	23,15	103
Seeds of soya	13,09	92
Red cooked beans	7,52	80
Cooked lentils	9,02	82
Baking soda	53,33	138
Miso	11,81	84
Hazel nuts	14,95	48
Nuts	15,23	48
Full egg	12,49	109
Pistachio	20,48	97
Split cooked peas	8,34	100
Chick pea	8,86	91
Pollen mixed	25	316
Quinoa	13,10	91
Wild cooked rice	3,99	74
Rye	14,76	71
Cooked soya	16,64	116
Dry seaweed	57,47	91

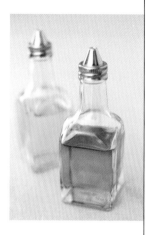

Don't give up with all fats

Be a well informed consumer, by giving the favor to unsaturated oils, by restricting saturated fats and not using trans fats.

Which oil to choose?

Let's take a look on the most usual ones and let's pay attention to fats acids available in each oil.

• **Ground nut:**

Contains 55%of oleique acid, 40% linoleique acid, 5% of a fat acid unsaturated.

This oil can be use in a moderate way for cooking because acid oleique is very stable with the heat. There is no alphalinolenique in it. So don't use it as oil for the table, you could do that only if you eat a very big quantity of nuts every day.

• **Rape (Colza):**

Almost no saturated fats acids. Contains: 50 % of oleique acid, 13 % alpha linolenique acid, 30 % linoleique acid. It's a very balanced oil, very rich in omega-3 and that's able to correct the deficiency in linolenique acid; a major problem of the modern food. This oil can be used every day more for the seasoning than for the cooking (don't make it smoke). It's also one of the cheapest oil.

• **Corn:**

60 % of linoleique acid, 30 % oleique acid, 10 % saturated acids. No alpha linoleique acids.

Mixed oils: Health or marketing?

Used to cook and to prepare seasoning, the mixed oils cannot contain, (according to the French law but not in Europe!),more than 2%of alpha-linolenique acid.

They are not so interesting for the ratio: omega-6/omega-3.

They are also expansive. They can be used for slow cooking.

This oil doesn't seem to be adjusting to a regular and exclusive use. Its big quantity of acids Linoleique stops it to be heated with a very high temperature. This could make appear toxics products (malondialdehydes).

• **Olive:**
85 % of oleique acids, 10 % linoleique acid and saturated fats acids. This oil can be used on regular basis, because acid oleique is good for health. It can be cooked but in a moderate temperature. But, as this oil doesn't bring any alpha-linolenique acid, it has to be use alternately with colza oil or to eat nuts.

• **Soya:**
Very few fats acids saturated, almost 70 % linolenique acid, 20 % oleique acid, 8 %alpha linoleique acid. This oil is less interesting than colza oil, but more good than corn sunflower oils, because there is alphalinolenique. This oil cannot be too much heated.

• **Sunflower:**
75 % of linoleique acid, 20 % oleique acid and also saturated fats.
Like the corn oil, this oil should not be the only oil of the family table. It cannot be heated with a high temperature.
To conclude, I advise you, to use regularly **olive oil and colza oil** (this one for seasoning).
Colza oil can be found in supermarkets. If you can give your preference to a virgin oil cold pressed. (you will find it in dedicated shops).

Special comment about the linseed oil

Trough the unusual oils, the nuts oil is a very good source of alpha-linolenique, as well as linseed oil (57 % of omega-3) or also oil of cameline (expansive).

The linseed oil cannot be sell in France because its stability is not high enough.

This defect could be easily resolved though a small packaging protected from the light and the heat, which is already done in a lot of countries, USA, Switzerland, Belgium…

Forget about recipe with fry oil and cooked oil

Everything fry, grilled or cooked in fry or broiling oil is absolutely politically incorrect!

All those ways of cooking bring toxics products. Learn to cook: steamed, or with Tinfoil paper in the oven and with a guide of dietetics recipes.

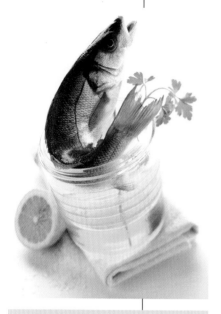

Full up yourself with omega-3

In order to increase your supplies in omega-3 eat fish and purslane!

We find omega-3 essentially in fats fish: Mackerel, salmon, harengs, cod, sardines. There is very few omega-3 in meat. Animals are direct sources of EPA and DHA, that's mean a long chain of omega-3 which comes into the composition of membranes.

Take a fish oil supplement

In the case of a lack of food supplies (not enough flesh and fish oils colza oil, nuts, soya...), those omega-3 can be bring trough a supplement of 0,5 to 2 grams a day of fish oil in pills.

Choose the wild fish...

Farm fish have a level of omega-3 much smaller (they cannot eat plankton, their source of omega-3). Caned salmon wild most part of the time, is a very good source of omega-3, when the fresh salmon of the Atlantic is a farm fish with 10 times less omega-3.

Pay attention to their concentration of mercury

Mercury exists in many different ways in the nature, but fish is the most evident way for the man. Predators fish like: sword fish, bass, shark, tuna, bonito, pick, have very high concentration in mercury. This seems to be, according to recent studies, a major risk of heart attack. For that for you don't have to stop to eat fish but you should prefer fats fish with a low level of mercury like the wild salmon.

Discover purslane

Purslane is the source the most reach in fats acids omega-3 from all the green vegetables.
In Crete, purslane is very abundant and grows in a wild way. Chickens are fund of it and also of insects and fresh herbs, those chickens give eggs full of omega-3.

Linseeds

The linseeds are an excellent source of omega-3. Grounded, you can add them to bread, salads, apple sauce, they will bring to those products a delicious and light taste of nuts.

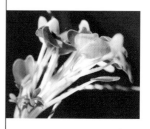

To make the long story short

The goods oils

For cooking: olive oil, colza oil, sesame seeds oil, fats of poultry. For seasoning of salads: Colza Oil, nuts oil, olive oil avocado oil, almonds oil, sesame seeds oil, linen seeds oil.

Oils to avoid

Sunflowers oil, corn oil, vegetal oil for cooking, margarine, heavy cream, fats particularly full of hydrogen.

Don't trust lights products...

They are all over the supermarkets. Unfortunately those products never helped anybody to slim down.
Let's take a look to the situation in America where the level of weight grows as the sells of those products increase!
To keep a good taste to those products, fats are replaced by agents of texture, modify starch, that's mean : sugars! They contain less calories, but "lights" products make us less full, less guilty also so we eat much more of them.

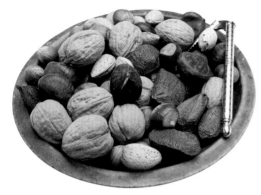

Nuts and seeds...
the health supply!

Our ancestors used to love them. Nuts and seeds used to be one of the major source of fat and energy when it was no other foods.

For those same qualities they are rejected today and could be even forgotten. They have a nutritional content very interesting. They are rich in **proteins** and **vitamins E**, one of the antioxydant the most powerfull.

Their fat are poly and mono unsaturated so, good for the heart.

They have a poor glycemic index. If you eat them with moderation (like 6 nuts a day) they will not damage your loss of weight.

• **Nuts of Grenoble** are the only one to bring fats acids omega-3 and omega-6 in almost ideals proportions.

Macadamia nuts are also interesting because they contains a lot of fat acid mono unsaturated (78,9 %), that's mean as much as olive oil.

• **Linseeds** are great for many reasons. They are very rich in fibers soluble and non soluble, they have very few pur glucids. Their glycemic index is almost zero even lower than most of the green vegetables. They are rich. They are rich in proteins and they have a lot of fats omega-3.

Quantity (mg/100 g) of sterols in some kinds of nuts and seeds

Cashew nuts	158
Almonds	143
Sunflowers Seeds	534
Sesame seeds non refined	714
Nuts of Grenoble	108

To fight against cholesterol, eat nuts!

Phytosterol are naturals substances that we can find in plants. Their chemical structure is close to the cholesterol structure. All the studies since fifty years shown that an important consumption of phytosterols bring to a reduction of cholesterol-LDL (bad cholesterol). We find those vegetal sterols in a large quantity in some oils like: olive oil 232 mg/100 g, sesame oil (2 950 mg/100 g) or wheat germ oil (1 970 mg/100 g). The refining of the oils reduce their contents in sterols from 20 % to 60 %. And when they are hydrogened, there is another lost of 20 to 40 %. Margarin is a bad source of sterols. For a good supply in phytosterols it's better to choose to have nuts and seeds.

Concentration in fats acids of different nuts

Nuts and seeds	Fats acids (%)	Fats acids mono-unsaturated (%)	Fats acids poly-unsaturated (%)	Alpha-linoleique acid (omega-3) (%)	Linoleique acid (omega-6) (%)
Almonds	8,2	69,9	17,4	0	17,4
Nuts of Brasil	24,4	34,8	36,4	0	36,0
Cashew nut	19,8	58,9	16,9	0	16,5
Hazel nuts	7,4	78,0	10,2	0	10,1
Macadamia nuts	15,0	78,9	1,7	0	1,7
Nuts of Grenoble	9,1	22,8	63,3	10,4	52,9

Nutritional value of nuts and seeds

Nuts and seeds (for 100 g)	Proteins (%)	Lipids (%)	Glucids totasux (%)	Glucids fibers (%)	Glucids purs (%)
Almonds	19	54	20	10,9	9,1
Peanuts dry grilled	26	48	19	8	11
Linen seeds	33	42	13	3,9	9,1
Sunflowers seeds	24	47	20	10,5	9,5
Hazel nuts	13	62	17	7,2	9,8
Cashew nuts	17	46	29	3	26
Macadamia nuts	8,3	73,7	13,7	9,3	4,4
Pine seeds	11,5	61	19	10,7	8,3
Nuts of Brasil	14	67	11	5,4	5,6
Pecans	9	71	15	9,3	5,7
Pistachio	20,5	48,4	24,8	10,8	14

Those nutritionals values can be applied to nuts or to dry seeds, non salted. Don't forget that it's better to look after the level of glucids purs rather than the total level of glucids: as it's difficult to digest fibers, only a part of glucids, the purs ones, will be absorbed by the small intestine and will give energy starting a production of insulin. The concentration in purs glucids easily absorbed is calculated like that: total level in glucids-food fibers.
EX: 100 g of almonds bring 20 g of glucids, but on those 20 g, there is 10,9 of fibers. So the level in glucids easily absorbed (20 - 10,9) = 9,1 g.

Control absolutely your supplies of sugars

The persistent excess of insulin responsible of the gain weight ,can be reduced only trough an appropriate diet which will exclude the sugars with an IG high.

The best sources of glucids are the one that our Paleolitical ancestors used to eat: fresh vegetables and fruits, not modified, rich in vitamins, minerals and especially of fibers. Those things have an average glycemic index, compatible with a diet program.

First of all take out from your food all the modified glucids discovered during the Neolithic time. Especially the sugar and the flour. All those refined glucids or modified help to gain weight, they bring unuseful calories for a very few nutritional and interesting elements. Also they create a vicious circle by giving a feeling of hunger when it's not even raging hunger.

The cereals

Practising the Paleolithic diet oblige you to accept to reduce your supply of cereals: **one slice of bread morning and evening, whole rice and pasta once a week.** For the others things…

- **With moderation:** grain of rice or whole wheat, whole oats, brown or basmati rice, whole rye, crackers rich in wheat fibers without sugar or fat added (like WASA crackers). Others whole cereals (quinoa, wild rice, etc.).

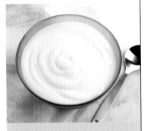

A snack for diet

You didn't have time to prepare your meal?
Use then a meal substitute rich in proteins and poor in glucids. Mix it with water only (no water, no juice fruit).

• **Not at all:** everything with white flower or refined seeds: white bread, sweetened cookies, waffle, crackers, pastries, croissant, white rice (beside the basmati), instant rice (to avoid completely), puffed rice or pasta composed with rice flour, white pasta (ravioli, macaroni, fusilli, fettucini), sweetened cereals. The others cereals to avoid are: millet, tapioca, corn, corn flakes, pop corn (same type).

Dairy products

• **With moderation:** Cheese <7 % of fat: once a week. Yogurt: 2 to 3 maximum a week, unsweetened, unflavored, plain with bifidus.
• **Not at all:** all kinds of milk drinks, sweetened yogurts and all milk products with sugar added inside.

Drinks

• **As much as you want:** waters rich in calcium and magnesium, herb tea, lemon juice.
• **With moderation:** sweeten drinks.
• **Not at all:** Juice fruit even fresh and without sugar added (they are too much concentrate in sugars, they don't have any fibers and very few vitamins). Cola and sweetened soda, lemonade, drinks with sweetened fruits and all drinks with sugar added. All alcoholic drinks beside wine.

Various

• **As much as you want:** All the spices and herbs beside ones with sugar added or with too much salt.

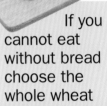

If you cannot eat without bread choose the whole wheat bread!

White bred doesn't have no fibers, no vitamins, no minerals and its' not so tasty.
In the whole wheat bread there is two times more minerals, until six times more vitamins and 3 times more fibers, precious for the intestinal transit, to balance the cholesterol and the blood sugar and to protect from colon cancer.

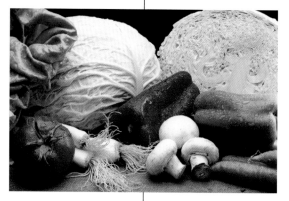

Fruits and vegetables for each meal

Compare to our Paleolithic ancestors we have the privilege to eat fruits and vegetable anytime during the year. It would bad not to eat them in abundance and take advantage of the goods things they are full of, then they are very tasty and their calories numbers are still reasonable!

• **As much as you want**

Fruits: fresh fruits as fresh apricot, avocado, cherry strawberries, redcurrant, blackcurrant,quince, raspberry, grapefruit, mandarin, mango, peach, pear apple, blackberry, blueberry, plum, nectarine…

Vegetables: All green vegetables, tomatoes, mushrooms, onions, artickokes, cauliflower and all things from crucifere, raw carotts, yellow beans, leek.

• **With moderation**

Fruits: To lose weight fast, in the beginning you must control your consumption of grapes, bananas, pineapple, dry fruits (figs, dates, apricots, raisin, prune) and papayas too much sweetened.

Vegetables: Greens beans, turnip, plumkin, cooked carrot, beet root, marrow.

• **Not at all**

Potatoe, baked ,mashed, fry ; canned fruits, jellies and marmalade sweetened.

During summer full up yourself with carotenoid

Carotenoids are the pigments who give the colours yellow and red and of a lot of fruits and vegetebales. Without them, **apricot, peach, watermelon, tomatoes, melon, peppers** would be sad to look at! The members of this big family: beta carotene, alpha carotene, lutein, zeanxanthine and lycopene.

Most of those substances are anti oxydant. Together, they protect our body from the permanent attack of the free radicals. This is accurate when those free radicals are numerous and abundant in some occasions: nicotine addiction, pollution and too much sun.

Interesting: lutein and zeaxanthine very concentred in the eye, are very efficient to protect from cataract or problems with the retina.

Winter time: Eat crucifere

The big family of crucifer has 400 members, the most populars are: **cauliflower, red and white cabbage**, Brussels sprouts, kohlrabi, curly cabbage, radish, black radish, turnip, colza, mustard and of course: sauerkraut (soucroute). According to epidemiologic studies, the consumption of those vegetebals help to reduce the risk of cancer (breath, prostate, bladder).

What kind of cooking?

It has to be different. Cooking reduce the value of vitamine C and vitamine B9 of vegetables. But cooking increase the lycopene, it's a carotenoide with an anti oxidant power very high.

To take the benefit of it and enjoy it, there is nothing better then to change the cooking ways.

Give more chance to steamed cooking or stuffed cooking without fats added neither sugar.

Fresh, frozen or canned?

If fruits and vegetables are known to be good and healthy, when they are not well preserved, some vitamins as vitamin C and E can be ruined. If you don't have time to go to do your market, choose then the frozen food because they better preserve all the vitamins rather than the canned food. But in an other hand, those one keep better mineral such as magnesium and potassium.

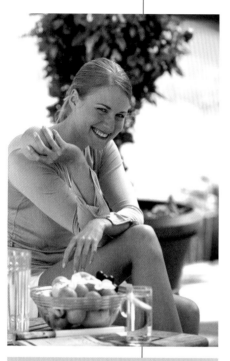

Looking for vitamins and mineral desperatly!

Fruits and vegetebales are the best vitamin and mineral sources. No one ignore that. But we eat much more less of them. Is that because their quality is not always at top and we had lost the sense of taste?

Real guardians angels

Fruits and vegetables contain an important quantity of micro nutriments very protective like vitamins C, E, B9 and A, or minerals like potassium, magnesium, calcium and also polyphenols. Trough all those micro nutriments, some of them play a particular part in the prevention of some diseases: vitamine B9, vitamine C, carotenoide, polyphenol and fibers have an action specifically against **cardio vascular disease**. All the micro nutriments with an anti oxidant effect prevent against risk of cancers, potassium protect from **high blood pressure** and **osteoroposis**.

To sulk the vegetables is that as dangerous as to smoke?

That's the conclusion of Dr Gladys Block (California University) after she watched deeply 246 studies that show that people who eat a few fruits and vegetables have 2 to 3 times more risk to catch a cancer. "It's especially true for lung cancers, larynx cancer, oropharynx cancer, oesophagus cancer, pancreas cancer, bladder cancer and colon rectal cancer. In a smaller way for the cancer of the breath, the uterus, the ovaries and the endometrium" the doctor said.

To avoid the vitamins loss...

• To choose fruits and vegetables the most fresh possible and bought daily. That's mean we have to eat as soon as possible our fruits and vegetables, like our ancestors used to that after they had pick them.

If you are lucky enough to have a garden, pick your vegetable few minutes before you will have to eat them.

• To eat fruits and vegetables raw rather then coocked. But think to clean them to take off any chimicals.

• Store fruits into the fridge better to let them outside.

• Use less water possible to prepare (the washing, the soaking).

• Peel and grate a little.

• To cook as quick as possible and avoid long cooking.

• Keep the water used for the cooking of the vegetables to make a soup. It's rich in vitamins hydro soluble.

• For vegetables the steamed cooking is better than the water cooking.

• To cook smartly and avoid the left over that will stay in the refrigerator or will be warmed again and again.

• The frozen products are more rich in vitamins than the canned food.

Choose the fruits and the vegetables from the Biological agriculture

The concentration of vitamins had been reduced since the big changes of the agriculture.

The use of chemical fertilizer, pesticides, the lands with a high return had empty the ground and plants have much less vitamins than before.

For that for vitamine E disappeared from the apples, the parsley, the lettuce and peas; same thing with vitamin B3 it's very rare in the strawberries.

Also we modified plants to increase their size and their sweetened taste. Let's take a look to the blueberry. The wild blueberry is small and contains full hand of wild berries to find the sweetness of two or three farm berries.

However wildberries give a quantity much more important of anti oxidant and nutriments.

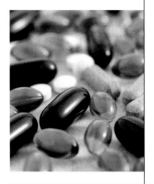

Do we have to take food supplements?

By following the prehistorical diet you are sure to eat more vitamins, minerals, essentials fats acids. But it doesn't mean that you will not miss some.

The selenium: Protection and detoxification

Very well known for its anti oxidant effect, this oligo element plays also a part in the detox of heavy metals (cadmium, mercurium, arsenic). The level of selenium of the elements depends of the concentration of this substance in the ground.
France and Belgium have a ground poor in selenium.

The vitamin E, The major anti oxidant

Numerous scientifics studies published since a lot of years came to the conclusion of the necessity to raise up the vitamins supplies in vitamines E, over the officials racommandations that say 8 to 10 mg a day. Those could be multiply by 3.
It was impossible those quantity in the food of today even eating more almonds.

We could think that to eat more healthy, as the prehistorical diet suggest it, we are definetly protected from deficiency in vitamins and minerals. Infortunatly some studies show that's not always the case. Why? Simply because the prehistorical man used much more calories than us.

With our 1 600 calories (Kcal) a day for women and 2 200 for men, it's difficult to receive the optimum quantity of micro nutriments. So that's why food supplements are interesting.

The anti oxidant

The prehistorical diet is very rich in anti oxydants, when we compare it to others kinds of diets. But environment had change since the paleolitical times. We are always exposed to toxics substances of various types which didn't exist only 100 years ago. The water that we drink, the air that we breath, most part of aliments that we absorbe contain left over of pesticides, chemical and industrial contaminant. It's seems impossible to escape from that. What is the long term impact of this exposition, no one knows specifically. But we

know better the excellent effects of vitamins anti oxidant and minerals on the disease related to the environment (some cancers, cardio vascular diseases).
You can choose a supplement anti oxidant bringing beta carotene, vitamin E, vitamin C, selenium, zinc. To take during course of treatment or for a continuous time. Ask your farmacist.

The Potassium

The prehistorical man used to have 8 to 10 g per day of it. It's 3 to 4 times more than today. Potassium prevent against acidose and rebuild the bounds. You can find in drugs stores supplements of bicarbonate of potassium (1 g a day).

Chromium

This element is essential to the metabolism of the sugars. It stimulate the receiver to insulin, allowing a better action of the hormone. But there is not a lot of it in our food. So it could be interesting to choose to have supplements of chromium (trough an organic way, biologicly active). To look for in drugs stores.
Needs:
- Teenagers and adults in a good health: 200 mcg/day.
- Men over 35 years until 400 mcg.
- People having an intolerance to glucose or to diabetese type 2: until 1 000 mcg.

Omega-3

Some people cannot understand to eat fish.
If you are one of them, don't hesitate to take daily fish oils in pills. They are rich in EPA and DHA, two fats acids omega-3 with long chains.
It's recommended for people in good health to have around 1 g per day EPA + DHA. We find easily those supplements in drugs stores.

The health benefit of fibers

The daily consumption of raw vegetables and fruits can help to keep a regular intestinal transit, because they are full of fibers.

The fibers effect

Fibers are essentials for well being and health. Because we don't have enough vegetables, fruits and oleaginous seeds and because flours are refined, we don't have more than 15 to 20 g a day of fibers, which is not enough at all. To obtain all the benefits of the different types of fibers it's recommended to have 30 to 40 g of fibers a day, choosing vegetables and fruits as main source of them.

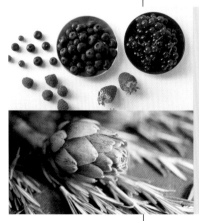

The best sources of fibers

There is a big quantity of fibers
in the green vegetables (artichokes, green beans, sprouts of Brussels, salsify, celery, fennel, endive);
in the red fruits : (Strawberry, Blackberry, raspberry, redcurrant, blackcurrant);
also in the wrack, a seaweed very reach in minerals which has a very stimulating action and known to improve the digestion and the feeling of satiety.

Others sources of fibers but less known: linseed and psyllium.

A fiber can hide another fiber!

Actually there is two kinds of fibers: fibers soluble and non soluble.

• **Fibers non soluble** exist as cellulose in whole cereals, vegetebales and rye. Because they blow themselves with water, they help to have a good intestinal transit, they prevent from constipation.

• **Fibers soluble** are in pectin (in the fruits), in alginate (in the seaweed) and in vegetable gum in some plants.

They absorbe big quantities of water to become thick solutions or even gels.

- They slow down the gastric emptying.

- They bring satiety and reduce the quantity of food absorbed.

- They reduce the speed of the absorption of glucids (and lipids) in the small intestine, impacting a reduction of the glycemia of the food (modification less brutal to the sugars absorption).

- They reduce the supply of calories: lipids are less well digested and almost eliminate in the stools (25 g of fibers retain 200 Kcal in the stools).

So by having soluble fibers (and also non soluble fibers in a moderate way) the glycemic index reduce, the secretion of insulin is smaller and we are less hungry. So you slenderize better!

The health benefits bring by the fibers

A cardio vascular protection

Some studies demonstrate that the mortality level trough cardio vascular disease is 4 times lower with people who have more than 37 g of fibers a day, rather than with people who have 20 g of fibers a day.

A protective effect against the colon cancer

If the part of non soluble fibers, (essentially in whole cereals), is not so sure anymore according some new studies, the nutritional research about soluble fibers are very interesting and prove their protective effect against the colon cancer.

The diary products

The milk and its by-products didn't exist in the paleolitic time (beside the breast fitting). Our ancestor could not milk wild animals! Today in France we have 140 kg of dairy products a year per person.

Say goodbye to ice cream, milk, butter...

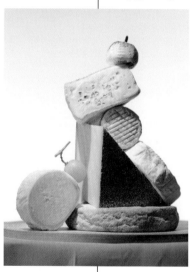

Here is the sentence. You will have at least in the beginning, eliminate from your food, the milk, the saour cream, the butter, which carry those saturated fats.

Those milk products could inter again step by step into your food. But they will always have to be eat in a moderate way.

Not more than 2 to 3 yogurts a week and cheese (poor in fats) just once a week.

Will I refrain my bounds to have calcium?

You will find good calcium in fruits and vegetables, in almonds, in fish, in mineral waters.

However you have to know that the mineral health of the bounds doesn't depends on the consumption of calcium. It depends also on the calcic balance, that's mean the difference between the quantity of calcium

Our milk: not good enough for the veal!

It could seems weird but veal never taste our pasteurized and homogenized milk. Those who touch it became sick!

absorbed by the body and the one which is execrate by it. A too much acid food create the leak of calcium.

To put back the acido-basic balance, the body is obliged to take calcium in its hidden reserve, that's mean : the bounds.

Salt help also to eliminate calcium in the urines.

Cereals, diary products, meat, fish, eggs produce acids actions in the body. The most aggressive ones are hard cheese which are also rich sources of calcium. On the opposite way, all fresh vegetables and fruits produce an alcalin charge in the body. If you don't have enough fresh fruits and vegetables and if in the same time you eat very acid food, you will damage your bounds and follow the road of osteoroposis.

By following the Prehistorical diet program you will burn 35 % or even more of your daily calories with fruits and vegetables alkaline which will neutralize the food acids bring by meats and fish. That's why we think that in this kind of diet, to bring calcium trough milk products is not necessary.

Food rich in calcium (mg/100 g)

Fresh sardines	290
Cooked spinach	256
Seeds of soya	255
Almonds	250
Schrimps	200
Fresh parsley	200
Nuts and hazel nuts	175
Watercress	160
Dry figs	160
Yellow egg	140
Cooked red beans	112
Cooked broccoli	100
Endives	100
Green olives	100
Cooked white beans	60

Mineral water is a good source of calcium

The tap waters are poor in calcium and magnesium they contain sometimes some bad substances (chlorine, pesticide, aluminium, copper). Choose mineral water which can also be used to prepare the teaand cooked the food which absorbed water like the rice. Through the waters the best in calcium and magnesium are Contrex, Hepar, Quezac, Rozana, Talians, Badoit, le Boulou.

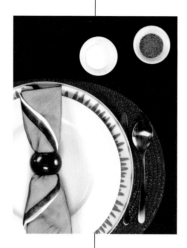

Don't add salt!

Our dish is defenetly too salted! Which has a lot of bad consequences on our health. This should push us to reduce our consumption of salt. Easier to say than to do!

Our far ancestor, even if they were not vegetarians, used to have a lot of potassium and no salt. The capability of the body to keep the salt had for sure, help the subjects to survive when they were able to keep this mineral. Many years Late, salt was used in a large way and this make excessive the availability in sodium and at the same time the consumption of sodium felt down. The various food modifications (white sugar, white bread) had empty the food from its potential of potassium. So the context is the opposite side of the situation of the first men, so the kidneys should keep their sodium and execrate in a massive way the potassium.

Not more than six grams

That's the quantity not to exceed, especially when we have a high blood pressure, obese or with have a cardiac deficiency. We eat 8 to 10 g a day of salt.
How? by eating: bread, crackers, cold cut, industrials soups, cheese, pizzas, quiches, mixed dishes, salted pastries, croissants, sauces and condiments and cakes and pastries. Those elements had been identified as being the main carriers of salt. They supply more than 80% of what we need daily.

We don't have any formal prove that the supplies high in sodium are bad for healthy people. However, it's better to eat less salty because this salt is suspected to bring osteoroposis, to increase the risks of stomach cancer and even to damage the cardio vascular system.

How to eat less salty

It's not so easy! Because it's not the salt that we spray on the food which is guilty, but the hidden salt contains in the industrial food. Excellent food preservative, flavor enhancer, it's improve the taste and the aspect of the aliments. For that reason it's always in our food.

Salt is everywhere even in unexpected places: chocolate, cookies, yogurts and milky desert, sodas. We ignore the accurate level of salt of those industrials products, because the labels give informations only about salt. Let's be reasonable and let's have less product rich in salt, let's pick fresh products, home made and let's try to salt in a light way our food.

Some tips to help you to reduce your consumption of salt

- Lose the habits to add salt to your food. At the beginning the food seems to be untasty, but after a while you will appreciate better their natural taste.

- Replace salt by other condiments, garlic, parsley, celery, onions, thyme, herbs of Provence, black pepper. Avoid mustard (too rich in salt) and a lot of industrials seasoning.

- Limitate the cold cuts,industrials meals, potatoes chips, salted butter, peanuts, aperitif biscuits, oleaginous dry grilled and salted.

- Wash the canned vegetables to take off their salt.

- Try not to put salt in the broiled water when you prepare rice or pastaor vegetables, because 30 % pass into the food.

- Some sparkling minerals waters are very reach in salt. Check on the labels their level of sodium (to multiply by 2,54 to obtain the level of salt). Replace sparkling water by regular water from the faucet!

Move!

To exercise regularly can have an important impact on your figure, your health and your energy.

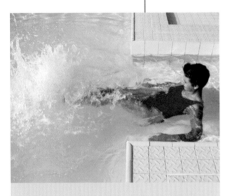

The aquagym to feel light even before you lose weight

This is gym in water!

Before our birth we had pass nine months in water.

So what is more natural for us than to move and exercise in an environment that we know so well.

With the ''Archimed push'' the submerged body is lighter, the tension of muscles is reduced and vertebras are reliefed.

This activity is particularly convenient for people who are overweight.

Important: it's not necessary to know how to swim to practice acqua gym!

Increase your muscular mass is a way very efficient to increase your metabolism and to allow you to burn more calories even when you don't do any specific effort.

Three kee words : frequency, variety and intensity!

To stay in a good health and prevent weight problems, it's not usefull to exercise a long time.

You can exercise less time, but in a stronger and intense way, your result will be even better.

That's mean that physical activity of few minutes but very intense and deep will have same effects than exercises long and with a middle intensity. But you have to practice more regularly at least 3 to 4 times a week the best being 5 to 6 times a week.

What kind of activities?

All type that you like and that will match your way of life: swiming, bicycle, jogging.

If you don't have time to practise regularly a sport, if you don't have a gym

close to where you leave, or even if you don't like sport, you can do some things like walk instead of taking your car, take the stairs and not the elevator, to clean the house every day!
Your body will react to effort becoming every time stronger and faster.

24 hours of an active day

For example, 20 minutes of a daily regular walk (with a normal rhythm), 30 minutes of house cleaning before and one hour of gardening will make you spend 800 calories.
To reach 1000 calories, nothing is easier: put some music on and dance!

Better to be chubby and active rather than skinny and sedentary

The Steven Blair group from the Alabama university in Birmingham had shown that the mortality of skinny and sedentary people is two times higher than active and overweight people (with an IMC over 27,8 kg/m^2).

Learn how to rest but exercise as much as you want.

To exercise or to practice a sport will never kill you if you don't take any forbidden drug.

Anyway we all be very tired before to accomplish enough sport in order to burn 9 500 calories a week.

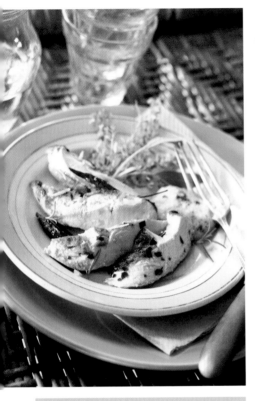

The Cro Magnon man passes us the dishes

Here some examples. Some prehistorical receipes to lose weight and enjoying food!

All those receipe are made are prepared without cereals, leguminous, milk products, salt, baking soda, refined sugars neither saturated fats.

Grilled cod with citrus fruits sauce (for 2 people)

Preparation

Mix the orange, lemon and green lemon juices in a bowl with the Cayenne pepper, the garlic, the olive oil and the water to obtain the marinade.

Put the fish filet on a dish and spill a quarter of the marinade on it.

Put into the refrigerator during 15 to 30 minutes.

Grill the fish during 3 to 4 minutes on each side.

Before serving spill the left over of the marinade juice on the fish, add chive and thyme.

INGREDIENTS

- 1/4 cup of orange juice
- 2 table spoons of lemon juice
- 3 table spoon of green lemon
- a few Cayenne pepper
- 2 pieces of peeled and crushed garlic
- 2 table spoon of olive oil
- 1/3 of water cup
- 1 pound of cod filet
- 2 table spoon of fresh cut chive
- 2 table spoon of fresh thyme cut thin

Scramble of eggs and spinash (for 2 people)

INGREDIENTS

- 2 spoon table of olive oil
- 1 pound of lean beef
- 3 chopped shallots
- 2 pieces of peeled and crushed garlic
- 1 coffee spoon of black pepper
- 1 table spoon of basil
- 1 cup of steamed spinash
- 4 scrumbles eggs

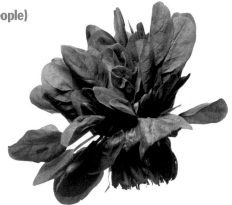

Preparation

Warm in a big pan the olive oil. Add the beef, the shallots, the garlic, the pepper and the basil. Cook it slowly.

Then add the spinash and cook it higher for 5 minutes and mix everything. Then add eggs and keep on to mix for 1 minute.

Veal liver in a Provencale way (for 2 people)

INGREDIENTS

- 1/4 of a cup of olive oil
- 1 red onion chopped
- 2 pieces of garlic pilled and crushed
- 1/2 table spoon of fresh basil
- 1/2 table spoon of rosemary
- 1 pound of veal liver
- 1/2 cup of Bourgogne wine

Preparation

Heat in a big pan the olive oil.
Put inside onion, garlic and rosemary.
Add to it the veal liver and cooked in a slow way during 10 minutes. Add the wine and cook during 15 minutes.

Roast bison in Bourbon sauce (for 8 peoples)

INGREDIENTS

- 2 kilos of roast bison
- 1 red onion chopped

MARINADE:
- 1 litier of red wine
- 2 big onions sliced
- 3 tomatoes, 1bouquet garni
- 2 glasses of Bourbon
- Whole Pepper, sweet pepper

For the choice of the pieces to prepare as stew, ask your butcher.

Preparation

Split the marinade on 1 kg of pieces of bison and put into the fridge for 24h. Mix time to time. The same day: drain the pieces of bison and put the marinade on the side. In a big pot warm, put the pieces of bison with the garlic and the onion sliced and the tomatoes. Add the marinade that you have filtered before, on coffee spoon of sweet pepper and some cumin in powder. Cover and let cook 2 hours and half in a slow way. Taste and check the seasoning if it's need to be modified.
To eat very hot.

Warm turkey salad (for 2 people)

INGREDIENTS

- 750 ml of mixed salad
- 250g of fresh turkey breast sliced
- 2 table spoon of olive oil
- 2 chopped greens onions
- 1 small sliced zucchini
- 8 to 10 cherry tomatoes cut in two
- Fresh ground black pepper

MARINADE:
- 2 coffee spoon of olive oil
- 4 coffee spoon of vinegar
- 2 table spoon of water
- 2 coffee spoon of Dijon mustard
- 1/4 coffee spoon of garlic
- 1/4 coffee spoon of pepper

Preparation

Mix the ingredients of the vinaigrette and put it on the side.
Put the salad on two dishes.
Cut the turkey in thin slices.
Warm the oil in a small pan.
Put the turkey in this oil for two minutes just to make them less pink.
Add the green onions and the zucchini and put that in the pan for two minutes. Add the vinaigrette and the cherries tomatoes.
Warm until everything is hot. With a spoon split the sauce on the salad. Put some pepper before serving.

Andalousian gazpacho (for 4 people)

INGREDIENTS

- 1 big chopped onion
- 1 pilled and chopped cucumber
- 1 green cleaned pepper cut in small pieces
- 1 or 2 pieces of chopped garlic
- 500 g of pilled and chopped tomatoes
- 1 table spoon of chopped parsley
- 1 table spoon of chopped mint
- Few almonds or hazel nuts
- 1 table spoon of oil
- 1 table spoon of wine vinegar
- 1/2 coffee spoon of sea salt and white pepper
- 1 litter water
- 1 cup of bread

GARNISH:

- 1 oignon cut in small pieces
- 1/4 of cucumber pilled and cut in small pieces
- 1 red or green cleaned pepper cut in small pieces
- 12 red or black olives sliced
- 2 hard boiled eggs chopped

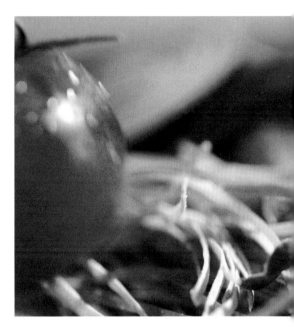

Preparation

Except the water mix all the ingredients in a small speed until you obtain a smooth cream.

Put the soup in the recipient and mix the water. Cover and put into the fridge long time before serving. When you serve you can put some ice cubes and add some Cayenne pepper. Serve the vegetal garnish on the side in small dishes.

Good appetite!

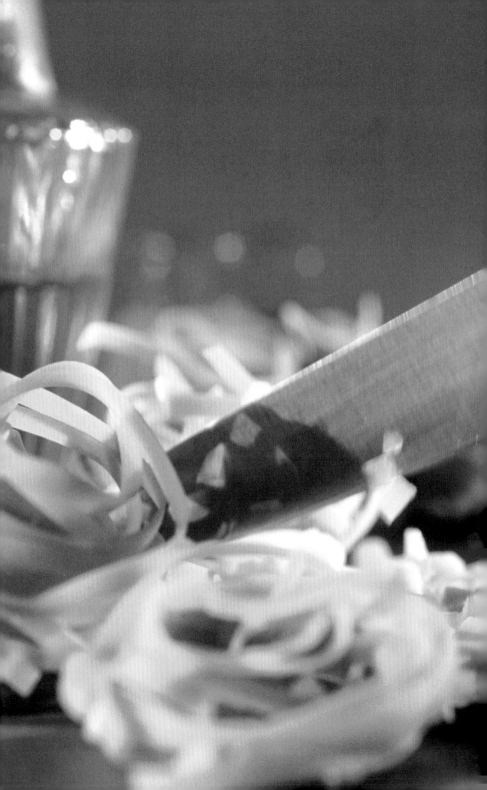

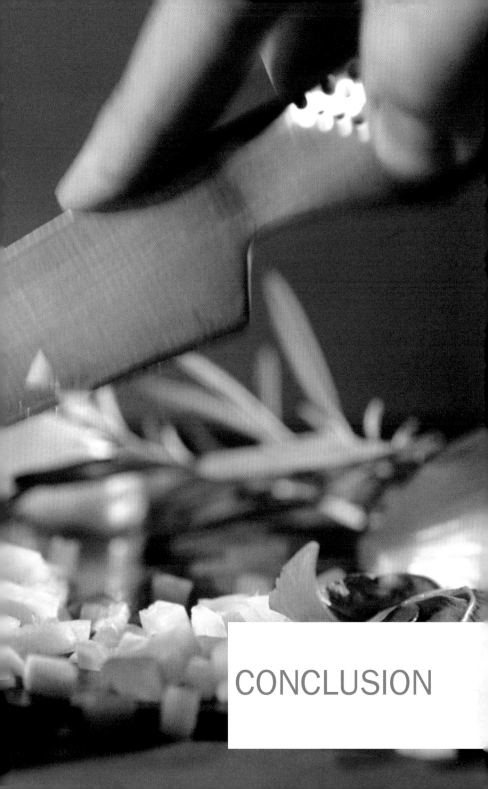

CONCLUSION

CONCLUSION

Let yourself guided by what mother nature offers us since man appears.

This include meat, fish, nuts, seeds, eggs, vegetables, wild berries and fruits, try to choose bilogocical products.

In others words everything raw and everything can be eated without being modified by technology. You could also reduce or even abandon the cereals (especially wheat) during a certain time just to see how you will feel (don't worry you will not face a food imbalance).

Food types	Green light	Orange Light	Red Light
Meats and substitute	Game, lean poultry without skin, All fish (fats) mollusk and seafood (shrimps, oisters, mussles, lobster) Goose, duck, horse, egg, ostrich...	Farm Meats (veal, beef, rabbit) Lamb and lean porc ,offal Lean cold cut (ham, Porc shoulder).	Pieces too fat Fish and fry and fried breadcrumbs fish Poultry with skin Fat cold cut (bacon, sausage...) And /or with too many additives and glucids (starch, flours, sugars...).
Fruits	Almost all of them: avocado, apple, Tomatoe, olive, apricots, berries, cherry, Peache, pear, kiwi, watermelon, melon, tropicals fruits, citrus and quince.	To lose weight faster Avoid: bananas, grapes, canned fruits (there is no vitamins in those).	Sweetened drinks, canned fruits in their sirop, Candied fruits, jellies and marmalade, Industrial juices fruits.
Leguminous			Peanuts, beans, lentils, cheek peas and peas.
Vegetables (fresh or frozen, raw or cooked)	Most of the vegetables are allowed: All greens vegetables, mushrooms, artichokes, califlowers, raw carotts, leek, yellow beans, aspara-gus, broccolis, beets, cabbage, celery, cucumber, eggplant, rhubarb, black-pepper, garlic, lettuce, spinash, onions, turnip, watercress.	Cooked carotts, beets, sweet potatoes, marrow.	Potatoes, gnoccis. To avoid completely: oven baked potatoes, mash potatoes, French fries.

Food types	Green light	Orange Light	Red Light
Diary products		If you can't leave without milk products choose Skim milk, plain yogurts and cheese with less of 7 % of fat.	Sweetened chocolate milk, sweetened yogurt, Cream and in general all diary products with added sugars.
Cereals		The cereals (wheat, wheat germ, barley, buckwheat, oat, rye) All those products must become a pleasant food to eat in a moderate way, in a whole way and without sugar, neither fat added.	Everything contains white flour or refined seeds: White bread, sweetened cookies, waffle, crackers, pastries, croissants, muffins, white rice and pasta, sweetened cereals. You must avoid others cereals like: corn, pop corn, corn flakes, millet and tapioca.
Fats		All fats. Nuts oil, olive oil, colza oil, sunflower oil. Home made mayonnaise using a good quality oil. Seasoning prepared with all those oils. Margarine non hydrogene, with sunflower oil or colza oil.	Peanut oil, palm oil, Butter, margarine hydrogen, mayonnaise, industrial seasonings.
Drinks	Waters, herb tea, lemon juice.	Coffee, tea, fresh juice fruits without added sugar, wine (red maximum 100 ml at the end of a meal).	Cola and soda, limonade, drinks with fruits sweetened and all kind of drinks with sugar added. All alcoholic drinks beside wine.
Various Others	All spices and herbs, vinegar.	Salt, mustard, chocolate with more than 70% of cacao. Sweeteners.	
Nuts and seeds		Almonds,hazel nuts, Nuts from Brasil, Pecan nuts, chestnut.	

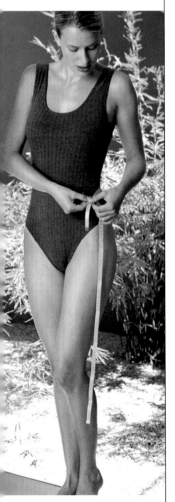

SLIMNESS:
THE ANSWERS TO YOUR QUESTIONS

To reduce the supply of certain food, as cereals or milk could that bring to nutritionals deficiency?

By following the tips of this guide, you will certainly eat much more nutriments than you used to do before. By choosing nuts rather than rice cake, fruits and vegetables rather than higly modified and refined nutriments, we absorb quantity of vitamins and minerals much higher.

From a nutritional point of view, food products to avoid are poor or they contain anti nutritional substances like cereals.

Is the big quantity of fibers bring by this type of food harmful?

If your fibers supplies used to be until then very moderate, it's important to introduce step by step, the fibers in your alimentation. And to drink as much as possible, water …of course! The large consumption of fibers on a short period of time can create abdominal pains and some flatulences.

To eat as much proteins could be a reason to gain weight?

No! The surplus of proteins cannot be stored. It's eliminated trough the urines. Actually proteins are absolutely needed and also in a big quantity in order to lose weight and escape from loosing the muscles (at least 1.5 g/kg of corporal weight a day).

Is an important consumption of proteins, as we advise it in this guide, dangerous for the kidneys?

Our far ancestors used to have plenty of proteins. They used to be healthy and didn't suffer from gout, as we can see it in the modern ethological studies. Only the people suffering from gout, important renal failure or bladder stone composed of acids uric have to watch their absorption of proteins. For the others peoples with no kidney problems, there is no danger.

We talk more and more about genes of obesity. The Paleolithic diet can fight overweight, but what about if we have those obesity genes?

Genes are an excuse! It's true that we discovered through serious studies, that several genes are related to obesity, like leptin or melanocortine, two hormons that control the sensation of satiety. For the same quantity of calories, some will gain weight, others will not! There is no justice in the nutritional matter.

However, fifty years ago the genetic inheritance of humanity was the same. And we would find less obese people. So, according to scientists, those genes don't explain the obesity epidemic, the food habits and the socials parameters have their part. The studies show that poor people who have an unstable food are more affected by obesity than other people.

I need to lose a lot of weight in a very small time. Will I succeed with this Paleolithic diet?

No. And this is not the goal of this diet which propose especially to modify the food habits on a long term.

Unlike the starving diets, the results are visible only after a few weeks. But once the lose weight dynamic will be on rails, your body will get use to burn fat and not sugar as a main source of energy and then the results will be obvious.

What is the difference between the Prehistorical diet and the others diets poor in sugars?

Most of diets poor in sugars are too reach in fats and they don't propose proteins. They also limitate the fruits and vegetables, which is a real medical mistake for health. So if those diets bring to a fast and important lose of weight, this lost damage the health and the well being.

At least but not last, it's only about to lose …water! On the contrary, the Prehistorical diet allows to lose weight on a long term, simply because the spends are higher than the energetic supplies.

A lot of food recommended in this diet (eggs, seafood, offal) are important sources of cholesterol. Do we have to exclude them to skip from an icrease of the blood cholesterol level?

For many years, the food cholesterol, like the fats, has been considered guilty about a lot of things. We have to mention a simple thing: Cholesterol is not a terrible killer poison, but an essential substance who helps the good functioning of the human body. Sexual hormons and cortisone, synthesis of the vitamin D and the bile salts: without the cholesterol, even the brain couldn't function normaly. It's indispensable that the organism produce a good quantity (around 70 %), when the food portion is limitate to 30 %. When this food supply is smaller the body is in a rush to produce some and vice versa. So despite the long time rumors, cholesterol food has only a small impact on blood cholesterol! The daily maximale dose in the food is around 300 mg,(according the OMS).

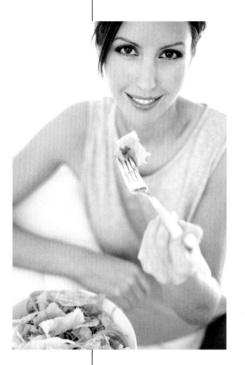

Some studies shown that to have 1000 mg of food cholesterol have a small impact on the level of blood cholesterol(around 5 %). Actually the main reasons of hyper cholesterolemia are: Obesity, a food rich in saturated fats, hyperglycemia constant (bad glucids all the time), a poor supply of in food fibers, too few anti oxydants, (vitamins A, C, E, zinc, selenium….), sedentarity, addiction to tobacco and stress.

By acting on those factors that we are able to reduce the bad cholesterol and also to prevent well and for a long time the coronarian disease.

Note: In general, people who have the Paleolithic diet have better blood levels (cholesterol, tryglyceridemia, blood pressure).

VOCABULARY

Acid alpha-linolenique: fat acid from the omega-3 family. It's an essential fat acid.

Advised daily supply (ADS) or nutritional advised supply (NAS): they are the exact daily dose of nutriments that we have to absorb to satisfy the needs of the body.
They are considered as a mark and not strict rules.

Allergen: Every substance able to start an allergic reaction.

Amino acids: Small molecule that form a group and become proteins. There are 20 of them. Each protein is caracterised by the number of amino acids which constitute them and by the sequence of those.

Anti oxydant: which fight against free radicals and protect from the oxydativ stress.

A substance guaranty: This mention means that the lost in vitamins and/or minerals salts existing because of the industrial process and the storage have been reward to establish the primary content.

Bacteria: element unicellular which is able to reproduce itself. They don't represent any danger for man.

Bio disponibility : the way that the body assimilate the food.

Calorie : Measure made of the quantity of heat needed to rease up from one degree the temperature of one grame of water. The food burned by the body give off a quantity of energy calculate in calories. To measure the energetic spends of the body or to express the quantity of a food, the results are described in calories (Kcal) or in Kilojoules in the worldwild systeme of calculation.
1 kcal = 4,185 kJ ;
1 g of proteins = 4 kcal (17 kJ) ;
1 g of glucids = 4 kcal (17 kJ) ;
1 g of lipids = 9 kcal (38 kJ).

Cholesterol : A compound from lipids that are in the fats and the animals tissue. It's furnished by food and it's in a part synthetize by the body. It participate to the constitution of the cells membranes. It's the precursory of the bile acid, the steroidale hormones and the synthesis of the vitamine D.
We have to distinguish two kinds of cholesterol: the good one (HDL) and the bad one (LDL). The first one have a protective part for the arteries.

Deficiency: Non sufficient supply from one nutriment or oligo-element needed by the body. It could be the consequence of a lack of supply or of assimilation of this nutriment or also an excess of lost.

Energetic needs: Quantity of food energy to give to the body as macro nutriments (proteins, glucids and lipids) to compensate the spends of energy. It's made of the basic metabolism (the enrgy needed to maintain the life of the human being during his rest) and the spends of energy related to thermoregulation, to digestionand to the muscular work. The energetic needs is not the same according to the weight, the sex, the age, the psysiological state (being pregnant, to breast feed) and the physical activity.

Essential amino acid: Element that our body cannot synthetize and must be bring by food. They are eight of kind: Insoleucine, leucine, lysine, methionine, phnyalalanine, threonine, tryptophane and valine. There is another one for the new baby born: histidine which is also essential.

Essentials fats acids: A fat acid is essential when it's essential for the future of a biological function, no matter which level (structure, biochemistry, physiologie). Omega-3 and omega-6 are concerned by this.

Fats acids: Elements which composed the fat part of food and the fats. The different fats acids are caracterised by their long carbon chain, by the potential existence of one or several double damage.
This bring to distinguish fats acids (no double damage), mono unsaturated (one double damage) and polyunsaturated (two or more double damages).

Food fibers: cellulose that is in the membrane of vegetals cells.

Free radicals: active molecules which can damage the cells. Factors predisposing to fast ageing and some disease.

Glucids: sugars or hydrate of carbon. They give the energy more or less quickly available.

Two kinds of glucids:

Simple glucids: they are in saccharose (in the sugar extract from the sugar beet or the sugar cane, in the honey, in the sodas), but also as fructose (in the fruits and vegetables) or lactose (milk).

Complex glucids: like starch, that can be find in cereals and bread, pasta, starchy food (potatoes) and leguminous (dry vegetables).

Glycemia: Concentration of glucose in blood expressed in g/l.

Glycemic index: the high of glycemia (level of sugar in blood) induct by digestion of a food compare to the one induct trough the ingestion of glucose.

Hormone: chemical substance produced by an organ (hypophyse, pancreas, thyroid) which react on another organ.

Insulin: hormone produced by the pancreas. It stimulate the penetration of glucose in the cells and participate to its regulation of its level in the blood.

Intestinal absorption: All the mechanism which allow the transition trough the cells of the intestinal wall of the nutriment in the blood or in the lymph circulation and from there to the different organs.

Lecithine: organic substance which emulsify (mixing water and oil).

Leguminous: Group of vegetables which the fruit is actually a clove (beans, lentils, peas, chick peas, soya, broad bean, ground nut).

Linoleique acid: fat acid polysaturated of the omega-6 family. It has eighteen atoms of carbon and two double damage. It's an essential fat acid.

Lipids: Fats.

Macro-nutriments: proteins, lipids, glucids sources of energy.

Micro-nutriments: vitamins, minerals and oligo elements protective of vital systeme.

Minerals: calcium, sodium, potassium...

Neutraceutical: It's a food-medicine. Actually it's an enriched aliment which have goods effects, (eggs with omega-3, milk fermented or yogurt with bifidus).

Nutrient : any and all nutritious substance which can be absorbed by the body

OGM: organism, genetically modified. Plant, animal, bacteria or virus in where we artificially introduce one or several gene. This give a better resistance to a disease, a higher level in sugar, a reduced sensitivity to the frost....

Oleaginous: seeds with oil. The majors are Sunflower oil, colza oil, peanut oil, soya oil.

Oleic acid: Fat acid monosaturated that the body knows to produce but that we can also find in the food, essentially in some oils (olive oil, colza…) and some fats (goose, duck).

Oligo elements: Essentials substances for the body, but in small dose. Some of them are very importantes because the body doesn't know how to produce them (cobalt, copper, iron fluor, iodine, manganese, molybdene, zinc).

Omega-3: Fats acids polyunsaturated from the alpha linolenic family, they are in some fish like salmon, mackerel and some vegetals oils (colza, soya, nuts).

Omega-6: Fats acids polyunsaturated from the linoleic family. We find them in most vegetals oils (sunflower, corn, ground nut, seeds of grape).

Peptide: Proteinic substances with a small number of amino acids (in opposition of polypeptides or proteins).

Proteins: Macro molecules made of peptide. They are the base of all cells alive.

Starch: Made of longs chains of glucose, it's the main reserve of glucids of the vegetals. It's abundant in cereals seeds, some dry vegetables and some tuber.

Starchy food: A group of products rich in stiffener: potatoes, cereals, leguminous, pasta, bread…

The digestion: A group of mechanisms physicals and chimicals of the degradation of the food to nutriments, which allow the substances and molecule easily absorbed, to pass the intestinal wall and to enter in the blood or the lymphatic vessels to be used or stored by the body.

Triglycerides: They are in our adipose tissues. They are made of a molecule of glycerol and three fats acids.

Virus: The smallest alive micro organism. They are able to reproduce by infecting another organism. Even antibiotics cannot fight them.

Internet useful

www.espritphyto.com
Online herbal medicine shop

BIBLIOGRAPHY

Bell SJ : *Low-glycemic-load diets: impact on obesity and chronic diseases*. Crit Rev Food Sci Nutr 2003, 43:357-77.

Cordain L : *The Paleo Diet*. John Wiley & Sons, New-York, 2002.

Cordain L, Eaton SB, Miller JB, Mann N, Hill K : *The paradoxical nature of hunter-gatherer diets: meat-based, yet non-atherogenic*. Eur J Clin Nutr 2002, 56 1:S42-52.

Delluc G, Delluc B, Roques M : *La nutrition préhistorique*. Ed. Pilote 24. Périgueux. 1995.

Eaton SB, Konner M : *Paleolithic nutrition. A consideration of its nature and current implications*. N Engl J Med 1985, 31;312:283-289.

Eaton SB, Eaton SB 3rd, Konner MJ : *Paleolithic nutrition revisited: a twelve-year retrospective on its nature and implications*. Eur J Clin Nutr 1997, 51:207-216.

Eaton SB, Eaton SB 3rd : *Paleolithic vs. modern diets–selected pathophysiological implications*. Eur J Nutr 2000, 39:67-70.

Eaton SB, Eaton SB : *An evolutionary perspective on human physical activity: implications for health*. Comp Biochem Physiol A Mol Integr Physiol 2003, 136:153-9.

Kopp W : *High-insulinogenic nutrition–an etiologic factor for obesity and the metabolic syndrome?* Metabolism 2003, 52:840-844.

Layman DK : *Increased dietary protein modifies glucose and insulin homeostatis in adult women during weight loss*. J Nutr 2003, 133:405-410.

Layman DK : *A reduced ratio of dietary carbohydrate to protein improves body composition and blood lipid profiles during weight loss in adult women*. J Nutr 2003, 133:411-417.

Ludwig DS : *Dietary glycemic index and the regulation of body weight*. Lipids 2003, 38:117-121.

O'Dea K : *Westernization and non-insulin-dependent diabetes in Australian Aborigines*. Ethn Dis 1991, 1:171-187.

O'Dea K : *Market improvement in carbohydrate and lipid metabolism in diabetic Australian Aborigines after temporary reversion to traditional life style*. Diabetes 1984, 33(6):596-603.

Piatti PM : *Hypocaloric high-protein diet improves glucose oxidation and spares lean body mass: comparison to hypocaloric high-carbohydrate diet*. Metabolism 1994, 43:1481-1487.

Rueff D : *Le régime paléolithique*. Jouvence, 2000.

Rowley KG : *Insulin resistance syndrome in Australian aboriginal people*. Clin Exp pharmacol physiol 1997, 24(9-10):776-781.

Simopoulos AP : *Evolutionary aspects of omega-3 fatty acids in the food supply*. Prostaglandins Leukot Essent Fatty Acids 1999, 60:421-9.

Simopoulos AP : *The omega diet*, Harper Perennial, New-York, 1999.